Chronic Obstructive Pulmonary Disease in Primary Care

Margaret Barnett

John Wiley & Sons, Ltd

Chichester · New York · Brisbane · Toronto · Singapore

Copyright © 2006 Whurr Publishers Limited (a subsidiary of John Wiley & Sons Ltd)
The Atrium, Southern Gate, Chichester,
West Sussex PO19 8SQ, England
Telephone (+44) 1243 779777

Email (for orders and customer service enquiries): cs-books@wiley.co.uk
Visit our Home Page on www.wiley.com

Other Wiley Editorial Offices
John Wiley & Sons Inc., 111 River Street, Hoboken, NJ 07030, USA
Jossey-Bass, 989 Market Street, San Francisco, CA 94103-1741, USA
Wiley-VCH Verlag GmbH, Boschstr. 12, D-69469 Weinheim, Germany
John Wiley & Sons Australia Ltd, 42 McDougall Street, Milton, Queensland 4064, Australia
John Wiley & Sons (Asia) Pte Ltd, 2 Clementi Loop #02-01, Jin Xing Distripark, Singapore
129809
John Wiley & Sons Canada Ltd, 22 Worcester Road, Etobicoke, Ontario, Canada M9W 1L1

Wiley also publishes its books in a variety of electronic formats. Some content that appears
in print may not be available in electronic books.

Library of Congress Cataloging-in-Publication Data
Barnett, Margaret, 1956–
Chronic obstructive pulmonary disease in primary care / by Margaret Barnett.
    p. ; cm.
  Includes bibliographical references and index.
  ISBN-13: 978-0-470-01984-9 (pbk. : alk. paper)
  ISBN-10: 0-470-01984-0 (pbk. : alk. paper)
  1. Lungs–Diseases, Obstructive.   2. Primary care (Medicine)   I. Title.
  [DNLM: 1. Pulmonary Disease, Chronic Obstructive–diagnosis.
  2. Pulmonary Disease, Chronic Obstructive–therapy.   3. Activities of Daily Living.
  4. Primary Health Care–methods. WF 600 B2616c 2006]
  RC776.O3B25 2006
  616.2′4–dc22   2005036664

British Library Cataloguing in Publication Data
A catalogue record for this book is available from the British Library

ISBN-13: 978-0-470-01984-9
ISBN-10: 0-470-01984-0

Typeset by SNP Best-set Typesetter Ltd., Hong Kong

Printed and bound in Great Britain by TJ International Ltd, Padstow, Cornwall
This book is printed on acid-free paper responsibly manufactured from sustainable forestry
in which at least two trees are planted for each one used for paper production.

Dedication

I would like to dedicate this book to all those affected by COPD.

Contents

Foreword

Chronic obstructive pulmonary disease (COPD) is a condition that is beginning to get the recognition it deserves. It now features in the general practitioners contract, has a National Institute for Clinical Excellence (NICE) guideline and the chief medical officer's annual report has a whole section devoted to it. Nurses are taking an increasing role in COPD management in all settings: hospital, community and in general practice. Nurses are developing skills and expertise that are often outstripping those of their medical colleagues. With the role comes the responsibility. COPD remains a difficult condition to manage well.

In the early stages, it is insidious in onset; the symptoms of even advanced lung damage can be attributed to ageing. It is striking how some patients with advanced disease remain very well, still able to keep cheerful and active while others seem to be brought down low by relatively mild disease. Each individual has his or her own response to the progressive symptoms dominated by breathlessness and the fear that attends it. Many are more crippled by anxiety than lung disease itself. As the condition deteriorates, breathlessness and lack of exercise combine to limit activities. By then, all that patients have to look forward to is the next exacerbation.

This book explains the process of lung disease, how to measure lung function and gives management steps. It also concentrates on practical ways to help the whole patient, including how to cope with the disease and control the feelings of panic and helplessness. Caring in COPD also includes the families, who also suffer from the limitations caused in the patient. Carers do not have a disease but sometimes it feels like they share the consequences, with loss of holidays, reduced social life and impaired relationships, including intimate relations.

Margaret Barnett brings her insight from great experience as a senior ward sister and as a community COPD nurse specialist. The first challenge is to make an early accurate diagnosis, which remains a problem with spirometry often being performed inaccurately. The importance of managing the patients effectively through all stages of the disease depends on listening to their concerns and providing the right information to enable them to cope with the disease in the best way. It remains the case that many patients fail to receive effective smoking cessation therapy, which could prevent their decline into disability. Nurses now need to understand the benefits of drug treatment and make sure that treatment is optimal. Nondrug treatments such as pulmonary rehabilitation are highly effective as they help all aspects of the disease. Patients unable to attend rehabilitation need to hear the messages about exercise and education, and promoting a positive view of living with COPD.

Throughout the disease process, there are things to be done to help patients. COPD is a great challenge, but is ultimately extremely rewarding.

Rupert Jones   MRCGP, GP and Clinical Research Fellow, Peninsula Medical School, Plymouth

Preface

This book is written as a resource for nurses and other health professionals caring for patients with COPD. Even though there are some 900 000 people diagnosed with COPD in the UK, the disease is still regarded as a Cinderella disorder and incites a negative image.

In this book, we explore the impact that COPD has on patients and their families and how we as professionals can help them to cope and improve their quality of life. It begins with an overview of the disease, symptoms, spirometry screening and clinical assessment of COPD. Alternatives to hospital management for acute exacerbations of COPD, such as 'Hospital at Home' schemes and their benefits are discussed. Medical intervention is only one approach to the management of COPD. A chapter is devoted to maximising the patient's quality of life in spite of his or her pulmonary limitations. The last chapter discusses end-of-life issues.

Since working as a COPD Nurse Specialist in primary care I have acquired a new understanding of the needs of patients with COPD as well as the support required of their carers. My role has enabled me to help patients who live a very frightening existence, to cope with their symptoms and make an impact on their quality of life. Caring for patients with COPD is both challenging and rewarding and I hope that I can pass on this experience to the readers to enable you to deliver the best possible care to your patients.

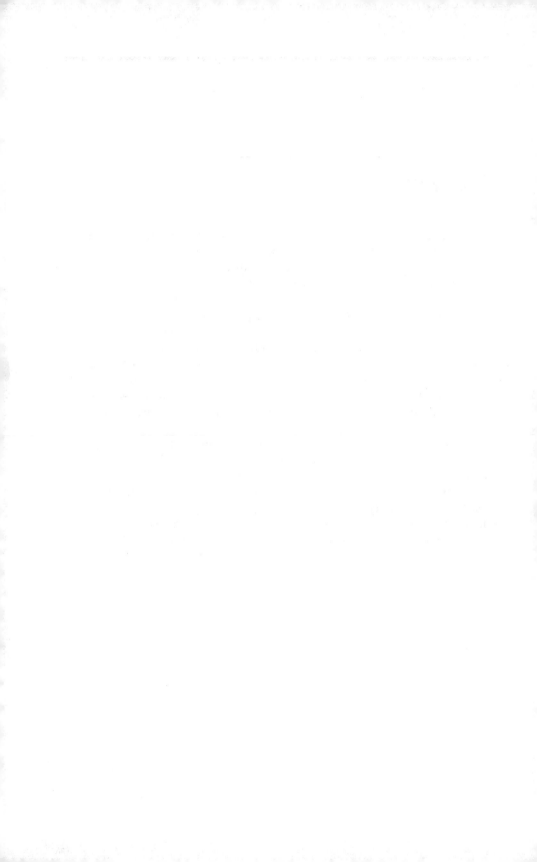

Acknowledgements

I would like to thank the following colleagues for proofreading the relevant chapters related to their speciality and for their support and advice:

Dr C McGavin, Respiratory Consultant, Derriford Hospital, Plymouth
Dr P Hughes, Respiratory Consultant, Derriford Hospital, Plymouth
Dr J Siddorn, Respiratory Consultant, Derriford Hospital, Plymouth
Dr Rupert Jones, GP and Clinical Research Fellow, Peninsula Medical School, Plymouth
Andrew Collingwood, Clinical Physiologist, Derriford Hospital, Plymouth
Jon Palmer, Ventilatory Nurse Specialist, Derriford Hospital, Plymouth
Jan Roberts, Macmillan Nurse Specialist, Plymouth Teaching Primary Care Trust
Russell Moody, Smoking Cessation Advisor, Plymouth Teaching Primary Care Trust
Christine Beer, Community Pharmacist, Plymouth Teaching Primary Care Trust

I am indebted to Sallie Waring, medical photographer, Derriford Hospital, Plymouth, for her major contribution in producing the photographs and figures. Thanks are also due to Dr McGavin and the following medical companies: Vitalograph, Clement Clarke and Boehringer Ingelheim for their support and permission to print photographs and illustrations.

My thanks also go to Dr Rupert Jones for kindly writing the foreword and to many patients for contributing their experiences and providing their permission to print their photographs. Lastly, my thanks go to my husband for his support and tolerance while I was writing this book.

Abbreviations

BMI	Body mass index
BTS	British Thoracic Society
COPD	Chronic obstructive pulmonary disease
CT	Computerised tomography scan
ECG	Electrocardiogram
FBC	Full blood count
FEV_1	Forced expired volume produced in the first second
FEV_1/FVC	Ratio of FEV_1 to FVC, expressed as a percentage
FVC	Forced vital capacity: the total volume of air that can be exhaled from maximal inhalation to maximal exhalation
GMS	General medical science contract
GOLD	Global Initiative for Chronic Obstructive Lung Disease
GP	General practitioner
JVP	Jugular venous pressure
LTOT	Long-term oxygen therapy
MDI	Metered dose inhaler
NICE	National Institute for Clinical Excellence
NIV	Noninvasive ventilation
NRT	Nicotine replacement therapy
$PaCO_2$	Arterial carbon dioxide tension
PaO_2	Arterial oxygen tension
PCV	Packed cell volume
PEFR	Peck expiratory flow rate
PH	Hydrogen ion
RV	Residual lung volume
TLC	Total lung capacity
VC	Vital capacity (relaxed)

Chapter 1

The Background to COPD

THE PREVALENCE OF COPD

Chronic obstructive pulmonary disease (COPD) is one of the most common chronic diseases in the UK. Most nurses during their careers will have been involved at some point with caring for patients with COPD. It is a major cause of morbidity and mortality. Worldwide, COPD causes about 3 million deaths each year (Bourke, 2003). In the UK in 1999, the number of deaths from COPD had risen to 32 155 (British Thoracic Society, 2002b), which relates to one in 20 of all deaths (Halpin, 2001), making it the fifth leading cause of death (*Social Trends*, 1995). By the year 2020 COPD is expected to be third in the rankings for the global impact of disease scale (Murray and Lopez, 1996). In England and Wales mortality appears to be greater in urban areas, with a particularly strong association with lower social class and poverty and higher smoking rates in this group.

COPD is a condition predominately caused by smoking and is therefore a disease that is preventable. It is a chronic condition that is insidious, and may not be diagnosed until the disease is fairly advanced with loss of 50–60% of lung function. In the UK, approximately 900 000 people have been diagnosed with COPD. However, the scale of this condition is probably underestimated, with as many as a further 450 000 people not diagnosed or mistreated as asthmatic, indicating that the prevalence of COPD may be much higher. Men are more likely to be affected than women, with prevalence rates of 2% in men aged 45–65 and rising to 7% in men over 75 (Bellamy and Booker, 2003). However, the trend is likely to rise in females over the next few years with the increase of young teenage girls smoking.

The total annual cost of COPD alone to the National Health Service (NHS) is estimated at over £980 million per year. Around half of this is due to inpatient hospitalisation resulting from exacerbation of symptoms. Costs within primary care are also high. In primary care it is estimated that an average GP with a list size of 2000 patients will have 150 patients with COPD, resulting in frequent surgery consultations and home visits. On average, patients with COPD have two or three exacerbations per year and treatment costs far exceed those with asthma, mainly due to the high cost of oxygen therapy. Within secondary care, COPD admissions account for approximately 10% of all medical admissions, resulting in over 1000 admissions per year (Barnett, 2003) per average general district hospital. The length of stay is also longer than other respiratory conditions, of around 10 days, adding pressure to an already overstretched service within secondary care.

Over recent years COPD has been largely neglected by health professionals and viewed as the 'Cinderella' of respiratory conditions. Many patients are seen as heart-sink cases with a self-inflicted disease, which is incurable and for which little therapy or medical treatment is available. The good news is that these views are changing, especially with regards to chronic disease management within primary care. COPD has therefore taken on a higher profile within the government and NHS agenda. Greater professional awareness has also been raised through the publication of the first set of COPD guidelines published in 1997 by the British Thoracic Society (1997b), which have had a major impact on the recognition and management of COPD. These guidelines have since been updated and released by the National Collaborating Centre for Chronic Conditions (2004) for the National Institute for Clinical Excellence (NICE), which are expected to enhance the profile of this disease further.

The government has at long last recognised that there is the need to manage long-term chronic conditions more effectively within primary care. The new document *Supporting People with Long-Term Conditions* (Department of Health, 2005) outlines a model of care for patients with COPD and other chronic conditions. Such intervention not only has the potential to reduce the number of admissions to hospital but also will certainly have some impact on improving the quality of life of these patients. Within various parts of the UK the Department of Health has set up COPD collaborative teams as pilot schemes to assist general practices not only to raise the awareness of COPD but also to enhance patient management within primary care. Along with this, the government made a commitment to modernise general practice and to tackle some of the key issues in caring for patients within primary care. In April 2004 GPs opted to accept the General Medical Service (GMS) Contract, which offered GPs and nurses the flexibility and opportunity to test different options for addressing primary care needs. The key part of the new contract is that GPs are paid on the quality of service provided to patients rather than the number of patients treated. This therefore allows practices greater freedom to design their services delivered to patients. Such a contract offers a greater incentive to practices to provide a first class service to patients, particularly with chronic diseases such as COPD. Practices are now required to record clinical data on computer databases so that audit of clinical practice may be performed and validated. Such data recorded by GP practices on patients with COPD includes:

- Accurate diagnosis of COPD
- Spirometry
- Smoking history
- Inhaler technique check
- Flu and pneumococcal vaccine given

DEFINITION OF COPD

COPD is a chronic, slowly progressive disease, characterised by airflow obstruction, which is predominately caused by smoking. The condition is not fully reversible and does not change markedly over several months. Airflow obstruction is defined as a reduced forced expiratory volume in 1 second (FEV_1) of less than 80% of the predicted value and an FEV_1 to forced vital capacity (FVC) ratio of less than 0.7 (FEV_1/FVC) (National Collaborating Centre for Chronic Conditions, 2004). Other definitions of COPD are shown in Table 1.1.

COPD is an umbrella term used to encompass chronic bronchitis, emphysema and chronic asthma. Chronic bronchitis and emphysema are specific

Table 1.1. Various definitions of COPD

National Collaborating Centre for Chronic Conditions (2004)
COPD is characterised by airflow obstruction. The airflow is usually progressive, not fully reversible and does not change markedly over several months. The disease is predominantly caused by smoking.

Global Initiative for Chronic Obstructive Lung Disease (2003)
COPD is a disease state characterised by airflow limitation that is not fully reversible. The airflow limitation is usually both progressive and associated with an abnormal inflammatory response of the lungs to noxious particles or gases.

British Thoracic Society (1997b)
A chronic, slowly progressive disorder characterised by airflow obstruction (reduced FEV_1 and FEV_1/FVC ratio) that does not change markedly over several months. Most of the lung function impairment is fixed, although some reversibility can be produced by bronchodilator (or other) therapy.

American Thoracic Society (1995)
COPD is a disease state characterised by the presence of airflow obstruction due to chronic bronchitis or emphysema; the airflow obstruction is generally progressive, may be accompanied by airway hyper-reactivity and may be partially reversible.

European Respiratory Society (1995)
COPD is a disorder characterised by reduced maximum expiratory flow and slow forced emptying of the lungs – features that do not change markedly over several months. Most of the airflow limitation is due to varying combinations of airway disease and emphysema; the relative contribution of the two processes is difficult to define *in vivo* (Siafakas *et al.*, 1995).

conditions, which present with distinct clinical or pathological features. There may also be some overlap with asthma, which if long-standing and poorly treated can lead to irreversible airflow obstruction (Figure 1.1). Some patients with COPD may also demonstrate an asthmatic component to their condition, with partial reversibility to bronchodilator therapy.

Other chronic lung diseases involving fibrosis (tuberculosis and sarcoidosis) or airway inflammation (such as bronchiectais or cystic fibrosis) may cause substantially irreversible obstruction or chronic mucus production, but these are generally not included as part of the spectrum of COPD (Halpin, 2001).

The term 'chronic obstructive pulmonary disease' (COPD) was introduced originally in the USA to describe individuals with varying combinations of airway disease and emphysema, and is now widely accepted in the UK and Europe. Previous terms used were:

- Chronic airflow limitation (CAL)
- Chronic obstructive airways disease (COAD)
- Chronic obstructive lung disease (COLD)
- Chronic obstructive bronchitis

However, the term COPD is a more accurate term as it is a condition that not only affects the airways but also affects the lung parenchyma and the pulmonary circulation in more advanced cases, leading to right-sided heart failure.

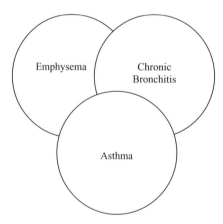

Figure 1.1. Diagrammatic representation of the three conditions that comprise COPD

PATHOPHYSIOLOGY OF COPD

Chronic Bronchitis

Chronic bronchitis is defined as the presence of chronic cough and sputum production for at least three months of two consecutive years in the absence of other diseases recognised to cause sputum production. In chronic bronchitis, epidemiologically the bronchial epithelium becomes chronically inflamed with hypertrophy of the mucus glands and an increased number of goblet cells (Figure 1.2). The cilia are also destroyed and the efficiency of the mucociliary escalator is greatly impaired. Mucus viscosity and mucus production are increased, leading to difficulty in expectorating. Pooling of the mucus leads to increased susceptibility to infection. Repeated infections and inflammation over time leads to irreversible structural damage to the walls of the airways and to scarring, with narrowing and distortion of the smaller peripheral airways.

The vast majority of smokers will eventually fulfil the above epidemiology definition. However, only 20% of this group will develop significant airflow obstruction (i.e. COPD). In the past these individuals have received the label 'chronic obstructive bronchitis' as opposed to 'chronic simple bronchitis'.

Emphysema

Emphysema is defined in terms of its pathological features, characterised by abnormal dilatation of the terminal air spaces distal to the terminal bronchioles, with destruction of their wall and loss of lung elasticity (Figure 1.3). Bullae may develop as a result of overdistention if areas of emphysema are larger than 1 cm in diameter (Halpin, 2003). The distribution of the abnormal air spaces allows for the classification of the two patterns of emphysema: panacinar (panlobular) emphysema, which results in distension, and destruction of the whole of the acinus, particularly the lower half of the lungs.

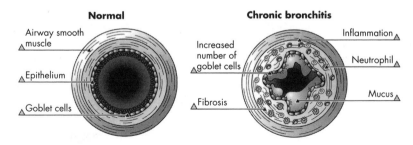

Figure 1.2. Changes in chronic bronchitis. Reproduced by permission of Boehringer Ingelheim

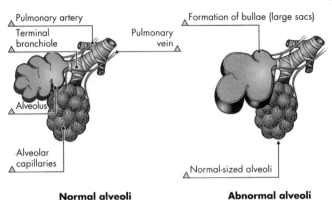

Figure 1.3. Changes in emphysema. Reproduced by permission of Boehringer Ingelheim

Centriacinar (centrilobular) emphysema involves damage around the respiratory bronchioles affecting the upper lobes and upper parts of the lower lobes of the lung (Bourke, 2003).

The destructive process of emphysema is predominately associated with cigarette smoking. Cigarette smoke is an irritant and results in low-grade inflammation of the airways and alveoli (Bellamy and Booker, 2003). It is known that cigarettes contain over 4000 toxic chemicals (Stratton *et al.*, 2001), which affect the balance between the antiprotease and proteases within the lungs, causing permanent damage (Crockett, 2000). The inflammatory cells (macrophages and neutrophils) produce a proteolytic enzyme known as elastases, which destroys elastin, an important component of lung tissue. Alpha-1 antitrypsin enzyme deficiency is associated with panacinar emphysema. It is the only known genetic risk factor for COPD, accounting for 2% of cases of severe premature COPD.

The alveoli or air sacs of the lung contain elastic tissue, which supports and maintains the potency of the intrapulmonary airways. The destruction of the alveolar walls allows narrowing in the small airways by loosening the guy ropes that help keep the airways open. During normal inspiration, the diaphragm moves downwards while the rib cage moves outwards, and air is drawn into the lungs by the negative pressure that is created. On expiration, as the rib cage and diaphragm relax the elastic recoil of the lung parenchyma pushes air upwards and outwards. With destruction of the lung parenchyma, which results in floppy lungs and loss of the alveolar guy ropes, the small airways collapse and air trapping occurs, leading to hyperinflation of the lungs. Hyperinflation flattens the diaphragm, which results in less effective contraction and reduced alveolar efficiency, which in turn leads to further air trapping. Over time this mechanism described leads to severe airflow obstruc-

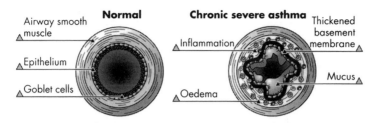

Figure 1.4. Changes in chronic asthma. Reproduced by permission of Boehringer Ingelheim

tion, resulting in insufficient expiration to allow the lungs to deflate fully prior to the next inspiration.

Chronic Asthma

Asthma is defined as a chronic inflammatory condition of the airways (Figure 1.4), leading to widespread, variable airways obstruction that is reversible spontaneously or with treatment (Bellamy and Booker, 2003). In some patients with chronic asthma the disease progresses, leading to irreversible airways obstruction, particularly if the asthma is untreated, either because it has not been diagnosed or mismanaged, or if it is particularly severe. Children with asthma have a one in ten chance of developing irreversible asthma (Rasmussen *et al.*, 2002), while the risk for adult-onset asthmatics is one in four (Ulrik and Lange, 1994). Studies by Agertoft and Pedersen (1994) and Haahtela *et al.* (1991) demonstrated in both children and adults how asthma might lead to irreversible deterioration in lung function if their asthma was not treated appropriately, particularly with corticosteroid therapy.

The airway inflammation in asthma over time can lead to remodelling of the airways through increased smooth muscle, disruption of the surface epithelium, increased collagen deposition and thickening of the basement membrane (Reed, 1999). This highlights the importance of patients being correctly diagnosed and treated to reduce the risk of long-term chronic obstructive pulmonary disease.

COMPARISON OF INFLAMMATION IN COPD AND ASTHMA

Asthma differs markedly from COPD in that there is a greater degree of reversibility of airway narrowing spontaneously and with treatment of bronchodilators or steroids. Although the mechanism of inflammation is important in both diseases, the inflammatory responses in COPD and asthma differ (Table 1.2). In the bronchial wall of patients with asthma there is a marked

Table 1.2. Comparison of inflammation in COPD and asthma

	COPD	Asthma
Cells	Neutrophils Increase in macrophages Increase in CD8+ T lymphocytes	Eosinophils Slight increase in macrophages Activation of mast cells

Consequences	Squamous metaplasia of epithelium
	Parenchymal destruction
	Glandular enlargement
	Increase in mucous production
		Fragile epithelium
		Thickening of basement
		  membrane
		Glandular enlargement
		Increase in mucous
		  production

Response to
  treatment
	Glucocorticosteroids have
	  little or no effect
		Glucocorticosteroids inhibit
		  inflammation

infiltration of eosinophils and CD4 lymphocytes, and degranulation of mast cells triggered by allergens in the airways.

In contrast, COPD involves inflammatory responses to oxidants in cigarette smoke. This activates airway and alveolar macrophages and epithelial cells. This results in recruitment of CD8 lymphocytes and neutrophils in the airways. As a result of increased levels of proteases and disturbance in the inflammatory mediators, mucus hypersecretion, extensive fibrosis and alveolar destruction occur (Hansel and Barnes, 2004). However, although we understand this pathophysiogical process and reaction to cigarette smoke it is not clearly understood why only about 20% of smokers will develop COPD.

Since inflammation is a feature of COPD, the effects of anti-inflammatory therapies would presumably have the same effect in controlling symptoms, preventing exacerbations and slowing the decline of the disease. However, the National Collaborating Centre for Chronic Conditions (2004) states that there is little evidence that inhaled steroids have any effect on the inflammatory cells present in COPD because neutrophils, unlike eosinophils, are relatively insensitive to the effects of steroids.

THE RISK FACTORS FOR COPD (see Table 1.3)

Primary Risk Factors

CIGARETTE SMOKING

Tobacco smoke is the main and most important cause of COPD (Figure 1.5). Although COPD can occur in patients who have never smoked, about 90% of cases are a direct result of cigarette smoking. Tobacco smoke is thought to

Table 1.3. Risk factors in COPD

Primary risk factors
  Tobacco exposure of more than 20 pack years
  Deficiency of alpha-1 antitrpsin

Associated risk factors
  Occupational exposure
  Dusty environments
  Pre-existing bronchial hyper-responsiveness
  Deficient diet
  Low birth weight
  Socioeconomic factors
  Childhood respiratory infections

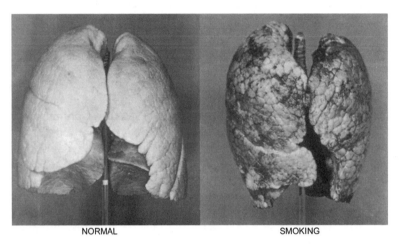

NORMAL   SMOKING

Figure 1.5. Slide showing a healthy lung and a lung of a smoker. By courtesy of Dr C.R. McGavin, Derriford Hospital, Plymouth

act as a bronchial irritant, leading to permanent changes to the mucus glands and to mucus hypersecretion. This results in the characteristic smoker's cough, which can evolve into 'chronic simple bronchitis'. Smoking also causes inflammatory changes in the walls of the airways and destruction of the alveolar walls, leading to the development of emphysema in susceptible subjects. Cigarettes are not the only culprits to cause COPD. Cigar and pipe smokers have a higher risk of COPD than individuals who have never smoked, although the rates are lower than for cigarette smokers (Hansel and Barnes, 2004).

It is also worth mentioning that marijuana (cannabis) may be a major cause of concern for the future. Although marijuana cigarettes are not smoked as often as nicotine cigarettes, marijuana smoking involves a larger volume and a longer breath hold (Vilagoftis *et al.*, 2000). Various studies suggest that marijuana smoking may not affect an accelerated reduction in FEV_1 (Tashkin *et al.*, 1997; Van Hoozen and Cross, 1997). However, a study by Johnson *et al.* (2000) reported a bullous lung disease in young adults who had smoked marijuana.

It is also known that there is a weak link between passive smoking and the risk of developing COPD. Smoking during pregnancy may be a predisposing factor for COPD for the child, as this may affect lung growth (Morgan, 1998). Young adults who have also had persistent exposure to parental smoking in childhood may have impaired lung function (Masi *et al.*, 1988) and are possibly more likely to have an increased risk of developing COPD in later life.

Fletcher and Peto (1977) in their study highlighted smoking as the most significant cause of airflow obstruction with accelerated loss of lung function that some smokers develop (Figure 1.6). As part of the normal ageing process from the age of 30–35 years, in a healthy nonsmoker the rate of decline of FEV_1 is usually around 25–30 ml per year, but in a susceptible smoker this doubles to around 50–60 ml a year (Fletcher and Peto, 1997). As the lung function steadily declines symptoms of COPD are not noticed by the patient until considerable lung function has been lost to an FEV_1 of below 50% of predicted values. Patients will usually present with symptoms of COPD between the ages of 50 years and onwards. If patients younger than this present with symptoms, then a referral to a respiratory physician should be made and further investigations other than spirometry should be conducted before COPD is made a firm diagnosis. In particular, a blood test for alpha-1 antitrypsin deficiency, a rare inherited condition, should be excluded as it accounts for 1% of cases of COPD (British Thoracic Society, 1997b).

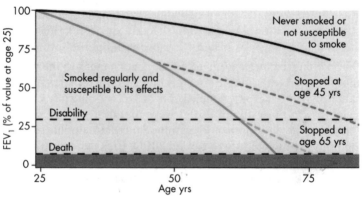

Adapted from Fletcher and Peto, 1977

Figure 1.6. Decline in nonsmokers and susceptible smokers. Reproduced by permission of Boehringer Ingelheim

There is a direct relationship between the amount of cigarettes and the number of years smoked, which is quantified in terms of 'pack years'. The formula used to determine this is

$$\frac{\text{Number of cigarettes smoked per day}}{20} \times \text{number of years smoked}$$

For example, if a patient smoked 20 cigarettes from the age of 17 for 40 years the formula is

$$\frac{20}{20} \times 40 = 40 \text{ pack years}$$

A smoking history of 20 pack years is a significant smoking history to contribute to COPD. We know, however, that for some reason a small percentage of patients with a heavy smoking history do not develop COPD. It is thought that this is because of natural differences between patients in the effectiveness of their enzyme-protective mechanism and possible other genetic tendencies.

COPD is more common in men (1.7%) than women (1.4%), which is reflected in the smoking of the past 40 years, and present with symptoms in their 50s and 60s. Of this generation a vast majority of their parents smoked and many patients will say that they were encouraged to smoke. Some will have started smoking as young as 11 or 12 years old and others were given free rations of cigarettes when they joined the Armed Services. However, many patients now state that if they had known the damage cigarettes could cause, they would never have smoked.

Patients diagnosed with COPD who persist in smoking should be encouraged to consider stopping. Although the existing lung damage cannot be repaired and the lost lung function cannot be regained, it is essential to emphasise to patients that it is never too late to stop. Fletcher and Peto (1977) demonstrate that by stopping smoking the rate of decline in lung function returns to that of a nonsmoker and therefore reduces the severity of COPD that may develop otherwise.

ALPHA-1 ANTITRYPSIN DEFICIENCY

This rare inherited condition results in the complete absence of one of the key antiprotease protection systems in the lung. It is a recessive disorder affecting 1:4000 of the population. Patients with alpha-1 antitrypsin deficiency are at risk of developing emphysema at an early age – between the ages of 20 and 40 years – and often have a strong family history of the disease. Patients with the deficiency and emphysema inherit one abnormal gene from each parent; that is to say, the parents are carriers of the gene. They will have half the normal levels of the antitrypsin in the blood, which may be enough to protect them from developing emphysema. Likewise, all the children of an alpha-1 antitrypsin deficient patient will carry one abnormal gene, but will not be affected. The two common forms of alpha-1 antitrypsin deficiency result from point mutations in the gene that codes for alpha-1 antitrypsin. This has important implications later in life for their children, who will carry the disease. If they marry another carrier, their children will have a 25% chance of being affected and developing emphysema at a young age. Although alpha-1 antitrypsin deficiency is responsible for less than 1% of cases of COPD, it should be considered in any young presentation of COPD, especially if the patient is also a smoker.

Associated Risk Factors

ENVIRONMENTAL POLLUTION

There is strong evidence that COPD may be aggravated by air pollution, but the role of pollution in the aetiology of COPD appears to be small when compared with that of cigarette smoking (Bourke, 2003). Air pollution with heavy particulate matter, carbon and sulphur dioxide, which are produced by the burning of coal and petroleum fossil fuels, are important causes or co-factors in the development of COPD. However, the Clean Air Acts of the 1960s have reduced industrial pollution although environmental pollution is still a problem. These are mainly from vehicle exhaust emissions and photo-chemical pollutants such as ozone, in particular, are to be blamed. Indoor air pollution from biomass fuel burned for cooking and heating in poorly venti-lated homes may be an important risk factor for COPD in developing coun-tries, in particular for women (Dennis *et al.*, 1996).

OCCUPATIONAL FACTORS

Some occupations where workers are exposed to coal, silica and cotton, such as miners, textile workers and cement workers, are associated with an increased risk of COPD. Exposure to cadmium, a heavy metal, and welding fumes has been recognised as a cause of emphysema since the 1950s (Burge, 1994). Coal miners are at particular risk and in the UK can now claim com-pensation if they fulfil certain criteria, irrespective of whether they have developed pneumoconiosis or have been smokers.

Many dusty occupations are more hazardous than exposure to gas or fumes and are associated with the development of chronic bronchitis and various forms of airway obstructive disease (Bourke, 2003). Shipyard welders and caulkers are also known to have an increased risk of developing COPD (Hen-drick, 1996), as well as those working in the construction industries who are exposed to cement dust.

CHILDHOOD RESPIRATORY INFECTIONS

Chest infections in the first year of life, such as pneumonia and bronchiolitis, may predispose to the development of COPD in later life (Strachan *et al.*, 1994). This may be as a result of incomplete development of the respiratory system at birth until lung growth ends in early adulthood (Stick, 2000). If developing lungs are damaged, maximum potential lung function will not be achieved, producing symptoms of COPD at an early age. A study by Barker *et al.* (1991) reported evidence from records between the periods of 1911 and 1930 of men born in Hertfordshire that showed lower levels of lung function in adult life among those who had bronchitis, pneumonia or whooping cough during infancy, and among those who had lower birth weights.

LOWER SOCIOECONOMIC FACTORS

There is a higher incidence of COPD in patients of lower socioeconomic status, particularly those living in urban rather than rural areas (Bourke, 2003). Within this group there is a higher prevalence of COPD in men than in women, where there is an increased incidence of manual labour such as mining and welding, which carry an increased risk of COPD. Smoking is also very common in this particular group of the population, but may not be the only causative factor involved. Evidence suggests other factors such as poor housing, damp conditions and overcrowding are likely to increase the frequency and spread of respiratory infection and raise the level of indoor air pollution.

Premature and lower birth weight babies are also more common among this group and have an increased risk of developing COPD in later life. This is possibly attributed to impaired lung growth *in utero*, through maternal smoking and exposure to passive smoking in infancy.

Poor diet is also another factor associated with socioeconomic deprivation. Low dietary intake of antioxidant vitamins (A, C and E) is associated with decreased lung function and an increased risk of COPD (Barnes, 1999). There is some evidence to suggest that a diet rich in fish oil is associated with a lower prevalence of COPD (Sharp *et al.*, 1994).

ATOPY AND AIRWAY HYPER-RESPONSIVENESS

There is considerable controversy regarding the influence of atopy and airway hyper-responsiveness as a risk factor in the development of COPD. These fall into two areas of debate. The British hypothesis proposes that the decline in lung function in COPD is due to damage caused by recurrent infection (Halpin, 2003), of which the pre-exacerbation lung function is never regained. On the other hand, the Dutch hypothesis proposes that lung function declines more rapidly in patients who smoke and who also have an allergic element (atopy) and raised levels of immunoglobulin E (IgE), leading to airway hyper-reactivity, as seen in those with asthma. It is known from early studies conducted by Fletcher and Peto (1977) that cigarette smoking accelerates the rate of decline in FEV_1, but it is thought that this may be greater in the presence of airway hyper-responsiveness (Tashkin *et al.*, 1996).

SUMMARY

COPD is a chronic disease of the lungs characterised by increased obstruction to airflow that does not change markedly over periods of several months. COPD consists of three conditions: emphysema, 'chronic obstructive bronchitis' and chronic asthma. Much of the airflow obstruction is permanent, although in some patients with an asthmatic component to their disease there may be some reversibility. COPD is a common clinical condition, predominantly caused by smoking. However, it may occur in some nonsmokers where occupational factors, atmospheric pollutants or an inherited tendency may be responsible for the disease.

Men are more commonly affected with this disease, although this pattern is likely to change in the future with an increase in young female smokers. It is estimated that COPD causes over 32 000 deaths per year in the UK and by the year 2020 COPD is expected to be the third most likely cause of death.

COPD is a major cause of morbidity and mortality affecting many individuals within primary care. By the time patients develop symptoms usually 50% of their lung function capacity has been affected, with much of the lung damage being irreparable.

Chapter 2

Presentation of COPD

PROGRESSION OF COPD

COPD is a slow progressive disease usually following many years of smoking, although other risk factors may also be responsible. COPD is rare in someone who has never smoked or has been a very light smoker. Patients will usually present to their GP with a history of increased cough and breathlessness on exertion (Table 2.1), which affects their mobility and quality of life. Initially, it is first noticed climbing stairs or slight hills when out walking. As the progression of the disease is slow, patients adapt and accept their breathlessness, thinking it is due to their age or being unfit. Most smokers expect to cough and be short of breath and either dismiss or ignore it as a 'smoker's cough', accepting it as normal, usually as a result of their smoking habit. Unfortunately, considerable loss of lung function may occur before such symptoms manifest and these patients therefore present to the GP when the disease is fairly advanced.

CLINICAL SYMPTOMS

Breathlessness

Breathlessness is the most common and troublesome symptom of COPD. It is subjective and is defined as an abnormal awareness of, or difficulty with, breathing (Bourke and Brewis, 1998). There are various terms used to describe types of breathlessness, as shown in Table 2.2.

Patients with COPD work hard to breathe in, and describe breathlessness in different ways. However, the most common descriptions are:

'I can't get enough air in.'
'The breathing tubes resemble a garden hose . . . . If you pinch the hose, it closes off. That's how it feels and you just can't breathe.'
'It feels like you're choking.'

Table 2.1. Symptoms of COPD

Breathlessness on exertion
Cough
Wheeze
Regular sputum production
Infective exacerbations
Fatigue
Ankle oedema

Table 2.2. Phrases used to describe types of breathlessness

Dyspnoea	Awareness of increased respiratory effort that is perceived as unpleasant or inappropriate
Tachypnoea	Increased breathing rate
Othopnoea	Breathlessness when lying flat
Hyperpnoea	Increased rate and depth of breathing
Paroxysmal nocturnal dyspnoea	Being woken at night by 'panicky' breathlessness

These phrases are what have been used to describe breathlessness by various patients. Breathlessness for these patients is a very frightening and distressing symptom and, like pain, can only be interpreted by the person experiencing it.

The descriptions given by patients are fairly accurate using their own terminology to describe the consequences of the pathological changes associated with COPD. Pathologically, the airways in COPD are narrowed and relatively fixed due to fibrosis and scaring, compared to those in normal individuals. Such airway narrowing leads to increased resistance and air trapping, which in turn results in reduced inspiratory airflow. As emphysematous changes develop, loss of elastic recoil and alveolar attachments of the lungs (guy ropes) causes the collapse of small bronchioles, making air entry more difficult (Table 2.3). Hyperinflation of the lungs with air trapping in the alveoli leads to an increased residual volume and as a consequence increases breathlessness on exertion. As a result of hyperinflation of the lungs, the natural dome of the diaphragm becomes flattened. This requires more effort to breathe, which places a burden on the accessory muscles during respiration. Consequently, any activity such as stretching up, bending to tie shoelaces or carrying shopping will worsen the breathlessness.

Although the airway obstruction has its main impact on expiratory flow, the effect of overinflation in putting inspiratory muscles at a mechanical disadvantage explains why, for many COPD patients, it is inspiratory effort that feels most uncomfortable. It takes much more effort during exercise for

Table 2.3. Increased respiratory work in severe COPD

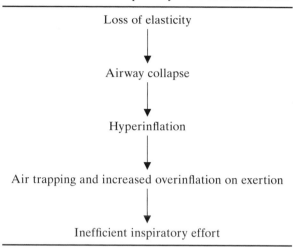

Loss of elasticity

↓

Airway collapse

↓

Hyperinflation

↓

Air trapping and increased overinflation on exertion

↓

Inefficient inspiratory effort

a COPD patient to draw in a breath than for a normal person taking in the same size breath. As the disease progresses, loss of the alveolar function in COPD makes gas exchange in the lung less efficient, leading to hypoxia as the COPD worsens.

Unlike asthma, the breathlessness of COPD does not vary markedly from day to day. However, breathlessness may vary according to environmental conditions and is often affected by smoky or dusty atmospheres. It is also sensitive to changes in the weather, particularly temperature and humidity.

Scales to Measure Breathlessness

There are various visual tools available to measure the degree of breathlessness. It is particularly important to accurately assess the patient's degree of breathlessness prior to any change in treatment in order to ascertain whether the treatment is effective. These tools provide an objective measurement and benchmark to which to refer. It is good practice to become familiar with the most suitable scale depending on the needs of the service you are providing to your patients.

MEDICAL RESEARCH COUNCIL (MRC) DYSPNOEA SCALE

The most widely used scale is the Medical Research Council (MRC) dyspnoea scale, which is recommended within the NICE guidelines (National Collaborating Centre for Chronic Conditions, 2004). This particular tool is graded from 0 to 5 and allows the patients to rate their breathlessness according to the level of exertion required to induce their breathlessness (Table 2.4).

Table 2.4. MRC dyspnoea scale. Adapted from Fletcher *et al.* (1959)

Grade	Degree of breathlessness related to activities
0	Not troubled by breathlessness except on strenuous exercise
1	Short of breath when hurrying or walking up a slight hill
2	Walks slower than contemporaries on level ground because of breathlessness or has to stop for breath when walking at own pace
3	Stops for breath after walking about 100 m or after a few minutes on level ground
4	Too breathless to leave the house or breathless when dressing or undressing
5	Breathless at rest

Table 2.5. Borg scale. Taken from Borg (1982)

Score	Degree of breathlessness
0	Nothing at all
0.5	Very, very slight (just noticeable)
1	Very slight
2	Slight (light)
3	Moderate
4	Somewhat severe
5	Severe (heavy)
6	
7	Very severe
8	
9	
10	Very, very severe (almost maximal)

It is an easy tool to use and record but each grade is fairly broad and may not be sensitive enough in some cases to measure the effect of a treatment.

THE BORG SCALE

The Borg scale is a tool that grades the degree of breathlessness from 0 to 10 (Table 2.5). This particular tool allows the patient to score their breathlessness according to the degree of breathlessness while performing a specific task. Due to a scoring scale of 0–10 it is fairly sensitive and reproducible.

OXYGEN COST DIAGRAM

The oxygen cost diagram is a visual scale, which lists various activities along a 10 cm line (Table 2.6). It allows the patient to mark along the line at which point their breathlessness would occur. The score is the distance along the

Table 2.6. Oxygen cost diagram. Taken from McGavin, Artvinli and Naoe (1978)

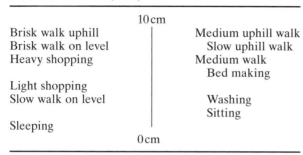

	10 cm	
Brisk walk uphill		Medium uphill walk
Brisk walk on level		Slow uphill walk
Heavy shopping		Medium walk
		Bed making
Light shopping		
Slow walk on level		Washing
		Sitting
Sleeping		
	0 cm	

line. This is a fairly sensitive tool in which patients may be able to relate a specific activity to their breathlessness.

VISUAL ANALOGUE SCALE

The visual analogue scale is another tool that can be used to assess the degree of breathlessness. A 10 cm line is labelled from 'extremely breathless' to 0 cm, indicating no breathlessness. The patient then indicates along the line the point that reflects their degree of breathlessness.

Cough and Sputum Production

In most patients with COPD, a productive cough often precedes the onset of breathlessness. The cough is usually caused by either irritation of the airway nerves due to release of compounds from inflammatory cells or by the presence of increased sputum production. Usually cough and sputum production in individuals who smoke is reversed once they stop. The cough is usually worse in the morning and is associated with chest tightness, which is usually relieved by expectorating. Sputum in such patients will usually be white and in smokers grey.

However, not all patients with COPD will have a cough and produce sputum routinely, except when they develop an exacerbation of COPD, which may become mucopurulent, yellow or green. Excessive production of sputum (more than an eggcup full) and frequent infective episodes may indicate a diagnosis of bronchiectasis and referral to a respiratory consultant for further investigations should be made.

Any patient with haemoptysis should be referred for a chest X-ray and a consultant's opinion. Haemoptysis can develop as a result of a number of reasons, such as a pulmonary embolism, tuberculosis, pneumonia, infective bronchitis, left ventricular failure or mitral stenosis (Table 2.7). However, the

Table 2.7. Causes of haemoptysis

Infective
   Pneumonia
   Infective bronchitis
   Bronchiecatsis
   Tuberculosis

Malignant
   Bronchial carcinoma
   Laryngeal carcinoma

Other
   Infarction
   Pulmonary embolism
   Pulmonary oedema
   Left ventricular failure
   Mitral stenosis

most important cause is bronchial carcinoma, particularly in patients with COPD with a history of smoking.

The production of large amounts of white or pink frothy sputum, particularly associated with increased cough and breathlessness at night, with orthopnoea may indicate left ventricular failure and pulmonary oedema.

Wheeze

Wheeze is caused by the sound generated by turbulent airflow through the airways. It is usually associated with asthma, particularly in patients with atopy and exposure to a specific allergen. In some patients with COPD wheeze may be evident during an exacerbation as a result of bronchial constriction. COPD patients may experience wheeze post exertion or when going out in the cold air or during windy conditions. However, unlike patients with asthma, patients with COPD are rarely disturbed at night with a wheeze.

OTHER SYMPTOMS

Chest Pain

Chest pain may be a feature of COPD related to intercostal muscular skeletal strain through coughing or intercostal muscle ischaemia. Other causes such as pleurisy, tumours or ischaemic heart disease should be excluded.

Frequent Chest Infections

Patients with COPD, particularly when severe or end stage, may present with frequent chest infections, especially in the winter. Symptoms of a chest infection consist of increased breathlessness, usually with a productive cough of yellow or green sputum. Wheeze may be evident in some patients at rest. Patients generally feel unwell, lethargic and have little appetite.

Ankle Oedema

Ankle oedema is often present during an exacerbation, particularly in severe COPD, usually as a result of the development of right-sided heart failure, otherwise known as cor pulmonale (explained further in the section 'Complications of COPD').

Anorexia

Loss of appetite is relatively common in patients with COPD, particularly during an exacerbation. This is due to increased breathlessness, cough and sputum production, which makes eating difficult and requires a great deal of effort. Loss of taste is also often common in these patients as a result of medication, in particular antibiotics and nebuliser therapy.

Weight Loss

Weight loss is a common symptom in patients with advanced or end-stage COPD, particularly those predominantly with emphysema. This is often due to an increase in the number of exacerbations per year and reduction in appetite. However, it is also as a result of a combination of factors, not just reduced calorie intake, but also the increased work of breathing due to their increased breathlessness. Insufficient calories are consumed to match the energy demands or metabolic rate required to sustain a steady weight. Other diagnoses such as lung cancer may also need to be investigated, especially if associated with rapid weight loss and other symptoms, such as cough and haemoptysis.

A low body mass index (BMI) and loss of lean muscle mass are common in COPD, especially in patients with emphysema. Weight loss is a poor prognostic sign and a low BMI increases the risk of death from COPD.

Fatigue and Depression

Fatigue is a familiar symptom in patients with a chronic condition, particularly in COPD. In advanced COPD breathlessness is a contributing factor in that the least exertion results in patients struggling to breathe. Various studies have revealed a strong correlation between fatigue, breathlessness and physical activity (Small and Lamb, 1999; Woo, 2000). This eventually leads to frustration, increased dependence and social isolation, which can result in clinical depression.

y

mptoms such as breathlessness, excessive coughing, frequent
rbations, fatigue and depression can have a huge impact on the patient's
qua.ity of life and daily activities of living, such as washing and dressing,
household chores or shopping. These things are taken for granted when fit
and healthy, but for patients with a chronic disease such as COPD, the sim-
plest of tasks can take several hours to complete. The assessment of such
disabilities is important to measure in order to determine the impact that the
disease has on the patient's everyday life. This will be discussed further in
Chapter 3.

COMPLICATIONS OF COPD

Cor Pulmonale

Cor pulmonale (right-sided heart failure) is caused by increased strain and
pressure on the right ventricle (right ventricular hypertrophy), secondary to
primary pulmonary disease. Increased pulmonary vascular resistance due to
hypoxia-induced vasoconstriction of the pulmonary capillaries produces
more strain on the right side of the heart. Eventually, this leads to hypertrophy and failure of the right ventricle (Table 2.8). As a result, peripheral
oedema develops due to right heart failure, which seeps fluid out of the capillaries into the surrounding tissue.

Anaemia

Anaemia may need to be considered as a cause for increased breathlessness
in patients with COPD, particularly if the patient has a poor nutritional
intake. A blood sample for a full blood count (FBC) will clarify this.

Polycythaemia

Over time, chronically low levels of oxygen in the circulation (hypoxaemia)
may result in an increase in the number of red blood cells. This is by way
of the body's attempt to adapt to the hypoxia and to produce more haemoglobin to carry what oxygen is available. However, one of the drawbacks
with this mechanism is that although it may increase the oxygen-carrying
capacity of the blood, it also increases its viscosity, with an increased risk
of deep vein thrombosis, pulmonary embolism or vascular event. The viscous
blood is also more difficult to pump through the tissues and this reduces
oxygen delivery. To avoid this, venesection should be considered if the
packed cell volume (PCV) is greater than 60% in men and 55% in women,

Table 2.8. Diagram to demonstrate the development of cor pulmonale

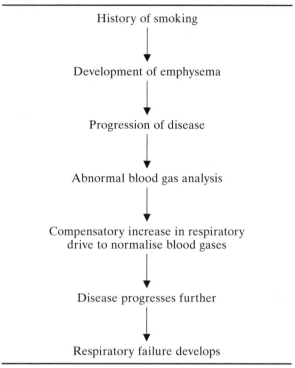

History of smoking

↓

Development of emphysema

↓

Progression of disease

↓

Abnormal blood gas analysis

↓

Compensatory increase in respiratory
drive to normalise blood gases

↓

Disease progresses further

↓

Respiratory failure develops

although the evidence for its benefits to reduce the above risks is rather limited (Halpin, 2003).

Pneumothorax

Pneumothorax may occur spontaneously in patients with emphysema. In emphysema the damaged alveoli form large air spaces known as bullae. These may rupture spontaneously, causing air to escape into the pleural cavity of the affected lung.

The symptoms of a pneumothorax include the sudden onset of pleuritic chest pain and increased breathlessness. A chest X-ray will confirm the diagnosis. Management will depend on the size of the pneumothorax. A small symptomless pneumothorax can be left to heal itself, a moderate first pneumothorax may be managed by needle aspiration and a pneumothorax over 20% will require a chest drain until the lung is reinflated.

Respiratory Failure

Respiratory failure is a feature of advanced COPD. Respiratory failure describes a state in which the lungs can no longer maintain normal oxygenation of the blood (Table 2.9). As lung function declines, the level of oxygen in the circulation falls and the respiratory centre in the brain triggers an increase in respiratory effort to maintain both the PaO_2 and $PaCO_2$ at normal levels. Eventually this mechanism proves inadequate to maintain effective oxygen levels, resulting in abnormal arterial blood gases. Some patients develop hypoxia but are able to excrete CO_2, known as Type 1 respiratory failure. In other patients the response to a low PaO_2 is impaired and their respiratory drive is dysfunctional, otherwise known as Type 2 respiratory failure (Table 2.10).

Table 2.9. Normal arterial blood values

pH	7.35–7.45
pO_2	10–13 kPa
pCO_2	4.5–6.0 kPa
HCO_3	22–26 meq/L
SaO_2	95–100%

Type 1 Respiratory Failure

This type of patient is usually very breathless, has a hyperinflated chest, is underweight and has a pink colouring, otherwise described as a 'pink puffer' (Figure 2.1). These patients have a well-preserved respiratory drive until the advanced stages of their disease with hypoxaemia and a normal or low $PaCO_2$.

Table 2.10. Classification of respiratory failure

	PaO_2	$PaCO_2$
Type 1	Reduced, below 8 kPa	Normal/low
Type 2	Reduced, below 8 kPa	Elevated above 6.5 kPa

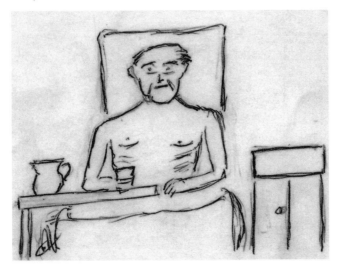

Features:

Breathlessness with pursed-lip breathing
Underweight – cachexia and muscle wasting
Use of accessory muscles of respiration
Hyperinflation with increased total lung capacity
No or minimal productive cough
Well perfused with fairly normal blood gases
Late onset of respiratory and heart failure (advanced stage)

Figure 2.1. 'Pink puffer' (good respiratory drive). Drawing supplied by a patient, Mr J. Young

TYPE 2 RESPIRATORY FAILURE

This patient has minimal breathlessness, has peripheral oedema, is cyanosed and is usually overweight, otherwise termed a 'blue bloater' (Figure 2.2). These patients have poor ventilatory drive often associated with abnormal blood gases with hypercapnia, hypoxaemia and right-sided heart failure, particularly during exacerbations.

Although the two distinctions of 'pink puffer' and 'blue bloater' are oversimplistic and not all patients may fit either pattern completely, they are useful in providing a visual picture of the two classifications of respiratory failure. An understanding of the two distinctions is important to remember when it comes to the management of advanced COPD, particularly if oxygen therapy is being considered.

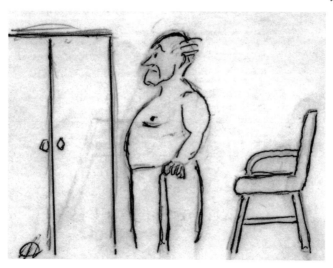

Features:

Mild breathlessness
Productive cough
Central cyanosis (blue tinge to lips, oral mucosa and fingertips)
Frequent infective exacerbations
Often overweight
Cor pulmonale with right heart failure – ankle oedema, raised jugular venous pressure
Respiratory failure – hypoxia and hypercapnia
Nocturnal hypoxia during sleep
Polycythaemia

Figure 2.2. 'Blue bloater' (poor respiratory drive). Drawing supplied by a patient, Mr J. Young

SUMMARY

COPD is a slow chronic progressive disease. It is predominantly a disease caused by smoking although other risk factors may also be responsible. Generally, symptoms of breathlessness on exertion and cough with or without the production of sputum present when the disease is fairly advanced. Usually by the time patients present to their GPs a considerable loss of lung function has occurred.

The natural history of COPD varies, with the two extremes of the 'pink puffer' and the 'blue bloater', although some patients may present with a mixed pattern. As the disease progresses other complications may occur, such as cor pulmonale, polycythaemia and respiratory failure.

Chapter 3
Diagnosis and Patient Assessment

INTRODUCTION

History taking and respiratory assessment of patients is now very much a role being undertaken by nurses in this field. The ability to undertake and document a clear, concise and systematic respiratory assessment of a patient is an essential skill, which enhances and expands clinical practice for those working within respiratory medicine. The various stages of history taking and physical examination will each be discussed in turn.

CLINICAL HISTORY

A diagnosis of COPD should be considered in patients over the age of 35 who present with a history of exposure to risk factors, particularly a long history of smoking, and who present with one or more of the following symptoms:

- Breathlessness
- Chronic cough
- Wheeze
- Sputum production
- Frequent infective exacerbations

During the early stages of COPD the patient will complain of minimal or no symptoms. However, as the disease progresses the symptoms will vary from patient to patient. Because of the insidious nature of the symptoms of cough, wheeze and breathlessness, patients with COPD often consider themselves unfit and unconsciously adapt their lives to suit their increasing disability. Smokers usually expect to cough and be short of breath and will as a result delay consulting their GP. As a consequence, these patients often present for consultation with advanced disease.

PATIENT ASSESSMENT

It is estimated that there are around 12 500 COPD patients per 250 000 (about 1–2%) of the population (Osman *et al.*, 1997). However, the prevalence is probably underestimated, with many patients not diagnosed or wrongly classified and treated as asthmatic. Therefore, to ensure an accurate diagnosis of COPD, it is essential to obtain a thorough history from the patient, followed by a physical examination and spirometry to assess the degree of airflow obstruction and confirm a diagnosis. In all patients with a possible diagnosis of COPD, a careful history should be obtained from the patient describing present symptoms and over what period these presented. For new patients an appointment time of 45 minutes is recommended for the initial assessment to be completed. Many outpatients or surgeries only allow 20 minutes, which is not adequate to complete a thorough assessment and establish a diagnosis and the impact this disease has on this particular group of patients (Table 3.1). A thorough assessment provides a benchmark for future assessments and evaluation of treatment and management plans.

Table 3.1. Aspects of history taking in patients presenting with COPD

Risk factors
  Occupational history
  Smoking history
  Environmental factors

Past medical history
  Premature baby, respiratory infections in childhood
  Other respiratory diseases: asthma, tuberculosis, pneumonia
  Cardiovascular diseases: hypertension, heart failure, ischaemic heart disease, atrial fibrillation, peripheral vascular disease, rheumatic fever
  Allergies/drug reactions, especially antibiotics

Family history
  Smoking
  COPD, asthma, bronchial cancer
  Cardiovascular disease

Drug history
  Current treatment prescribed for COPD
  Other medication taken, particularly beta-blockers
  Over-the-counter drugs taken
  Herbal remedies
  Vaccination status

Social history
  Home conditions
  Social and family support
  Impact of disease on patient's daily activities of living: mobility, washing and dressing, hobbies and social interaction
  Diet and alcohol consumption

PATIENT HISTORY

Risk Factors

A patient's occupation and exposure to risk factors such as occupational or environmental factors are important. A detailed history of tobacco usage should be obtained (preferably not one of the first things asked), including the number of years and number of cigarettes smoked. Smoking of a pipe or cigars should also be noted. A significant smoking history for COPD is more than 15–20 pack years. If the smoking history if much less with little exposure to other risk factors an alternative diagnosis may need to be investigated.

Medical History

Start by asking the patient if they have any medical problems. Past medical history including asthma, allergies, sinusitis or nasal polyps, previous childhood respiratory infections or other respiratory diseases such as tuberculosis or pneumonia are important to differentiate a diagnosis.

The presence of co-morbidities, such as heart disease, hypertension and arthritis, may contribute to restriction of activity. The pattern of symptom development relating to breathlessness, cough, wheeze and the production of sputum, and over what time scale, is beneficial, to help confirm the diagnosis and to rule out other diagnoses. A history of previous exacerbations and frequency is useful. Patients may be more aware of periods when their symptoms were worse, particularly during the winter months.

Family History

This is taken to obtain information about the patient's blood relatives (grandparents, parents, siblings and children). In particular, questions related to inheritable diseases are important here. Most common are illnesses such as other chronic respiratory disease, COPD, asthma or lung cancer, as well as cardiovascular disease, such as ischaemic heart disease (angina and a history of myocardial infarctions). It is also essential to find out the age of onset of the illness, as this may be of prognostic importance for the patient. Also seek information about any unusual illnesses among the family, which may reveal evidence of rare genetic conditions. For example, if a young patient (20–40 years) presents with breathlessness and reduced lung function with a family history of smoking and emphysema, alpha-1 antitrypsin deficiency would need to be excluded.

Drug History

Details of the patient's current drug management and compliance are important to determine, in particular dose and frequency. Confusion about or noncompliance with medication is a big problem in many elderly patients, especially if the drug regimens are complex. Therefore, it is important to actually go through all the patient's medication to ascertain if he or she is actually taking the medication as prescribed. Just glancing at a list of medication the patient produces or a copy of the patient's repeat prescription list is not really adequate. It is useful to request the patient to actually bring all the medication to the clinic or ask the patient to have them ready to show you when you visit his or her home. In particular, appropriateness of respiratory therapy such as inhaled or nebulised therapy is important. This can provide critical information, as frequently what appears to be a failure to respond to a particular therapy may actually be related to noncompliance for one reason or another. Beta-adrenergic antagonists ('beta-blockers') are commonly prescribed in this age group for hypertension and angina, and as eye drops for glaucoma. These drugs are contraindicated in COPD as they aggravate airflow obstruction and interfere with the action of agonists such as salbutamol. It is therefore really important to have a good knowledge of all drugs patients in your care have been prescribed, and their side effects as well as contraindications. In addition to prescribed medication, patients should be asked if they are taking any over-the-counter drugs or herbal remedies, the amount and the reason they take them.

Details of vaccination against influenza and *Streptococcus pneumoniae* (Pnumovax) should be recorded.

Known Allergies/Drug Reactions

It is important to ascertain if the patient has any drug allergies or any adverse reactions to any medication. The exact nature of the reaction should be clearly identified as it can have important clinical implications such as anaphylaxis, which is a life-threatening reaction. Most reactions, however, usually appear as a rash. Such information should be clearly documented in the patient's records and the patient made aware that any drugs that produce a reaction should be avoided.

Social History

Information regarding home conditions and family support is significant to establish how the patient copes at home. It is useful to know the general layout of the home, such as whether he or she lives on one level or has stairs or steps to the accommodation, as well as indoors, and if rails are in position to provide some assistance. If the patient lives in a block of flats, is there access to a lift and if not how many flights of stairs have to be climbed? If patients have difficulty climbing stairs/steps this may be the reason why some patients become house bound and do not go out. If this is the reason and they live in council properties maybe they could consider a transfer to a property with easier access or on one level.

It is useful to know what family support these patients have. Do they live on their own or with a spouse or partner? Do they have regular visits from family or friends? Are they receiving any support from Age Concern or social services, such as home care, meals on wheels or help with their housework? Are they receiving any form of benefits that they may be entitled to?

IMPACT OF THE DISEASE ON DAILY LIVING

Close questioning about the patient's ability to perform tasks related to daily activities of living is required in order to assess the impact of the disease on daily life. It is important that the health professional asks specific and detailed questions to establish a clear picture of each individual patient's routine and activities. Health professionals are in a unique position to assess the true impact this debilitating disease has on the patient's and carer's daily lives. Only by taking time to obtain this information will you, as health professionals, be able to make a real difference to their lives in terms of providing effective education, support and drug management.

To obtain a concise assessment of the impact this disease has on individual patients it is useful to use some form of nursing model as a form of framework. There are many well-known nursing models that have been devised over the years. Ultimately the main concepts shared by nursing models are related to the patient, environment, health and nursing activities (Roper, Logan and Tierney, 2001). Orem's 'self-care' depicts nursing as assisting the patient to an optimal level of self-care (Orem, 1971). Roy (1970) centred her model on the concept of adaptation. Rogers (1970) focused on the concept of the environment and the patient in interaction with the environment. However, the Roper, Logan and Tierney (2000) nursing model is recommended, as it is easy to understand and apply to this particular group of patients and covers all aspects of daily living (Table 3.2). It provides a suitable framework for the patient's physical abilities and needs, while highlighting areas of care to promote patient independence. Roper's model also applies a problem-solving approach in the assessment and management of patients with COPD: assess, plan, implement and evaluate individual patient care. The model is based on 12 activities of daily living as outlined below, which relate to either essential functions for the maintenance of life (i.e. breathing, eating, sleeping, eliminating) or others to increase the quality of life (i.e. communicating, washing, dressing, working, learning). Of course it is not only essential to establish any difficulties the patient may be experiencing with any daily activities of living, but also to discuss and plan how these problems may be addressed. This will invariably require contacting members of the multidisciplinary team/outside agencies for further assessment and assistance.

Table 3.2. Impact of disease on daily living using the Roper, Hogan and Tierney (2000) model of nursing

Activities of daily living	Patient assessment
1. Maintaining a safe environment	
2. Communication	
3. Breathing	
4. Mobility	
5. Hygiene needs and dressing	
6. Nutrition	
7. Elimination	
8. Sleeping	
9. Expressing sexuality	
10. Social activities	
11. Working and playing	
12. Dying	

1. Maintaining a Safe Environment

Establish some information regarding patients' home circumstances and home conditions. Questions to ask:

- Do they live on one level?
- Do they have steps outside to access their home?
- Do they have to use the stairs or have they a stair lift installed which they have to access to go up to bed or to use the bathroom? Do they have a toilet downstairs?
- What type of heating do they have?

It is essential to ascertain the type of environment in which the patient lives and to ensure that it is safe, as many patients are elderly. Every precaution should therefore be taken to prevent accidents and falls. This includes the availability of aids or rails to assist with mobility in order to maintain their independence. Referral to other members of the multidisciplinary team such as the occupational therapist, physiotherapist or social worker may be necessary for further assessment.

2. Communication

Questions to ask:

- Do they have any hearing or sight impairment?
- Do they have any difficulty in talking (i.e. due to a stroke) or understanding your language?
- Do they have difficulty in reading or writing?

Communication is an essential activity and an integral part of all human behaviour. It does not just relate to speech but involves other sensory perception such as seeing and hearing, as well as nonverbal communication. All these factors will affect the health professional's and patient's ability to communicate with each other effectively. Methods will need to be developed to address any difficulties, as this may affect the initial assessment and the patient's compliance with new treatment. If hearing or sight is a particular problem further referral to an appropriate specialist or therapist may be required.

3. Breathing

Questions to ask:

- What activities cause patients to be breathless (i.e. bending, stretching, eating, getting out of a chair)?
- Are there any symptoms that cause breathlessness such as coughing or difficulty in expectorating sputum?
- Do they suffer from panic/anxiety attacks? If so, when do they occur and how often?

Breathing is an activity our body is dependent on to maintain life itself. For an individual without COPD breathing is an effortless activity that subconsciously we are not aware of performing. However, for most patients with this condition, particularly those with severe COPD, every breath can be a struggle. It is important to establish whether the patients are breathless following an activity and how long it takes for them to recover. What positions do patients adopt to help them recover? Do they need to use an inhaler or oxygen to help them recover? Do they suffer from panic attacks if they get breathless and, if so, how do they cope? There are various breathless assessment tools available (Table 3.3), which will be discussed further in Chapter 4.

4. Mobility

Questions to ask:

- Do the patients have problems with mobility?
- How far can they walk on the flat without stopping?
- Do they find going up slight inclines or steps difficult because of their breathing?
- Do they use some form of walking aid when mobilising?
- What difficulties do patients feel they have with mobility and how do they cope?

Table 3.3. Breathlessness assessment tools

Test	Description of tool
MRC breathlessness score (Fletcher *et al.*, 1959)	Patients grade activities (1–5) according to degree of breathlessness
Borg scale (Borg, 1982)	Patients grade their breathlessness during a particular activity (0–10)
Oxygen cost diagram (McGavin, Artvinli and Naoe, 1978)	The diagram lists various activities along a 10 cm line. The patient marks at which point breathlessness would occur. The score is the distance along the line
Visual analogue scale (Noseda, Capreiaux and Schmerber, 1992)	The patient indicates along a line of 10 cm, which is marked 'no breathlessness' at 0 cm, and 'extremely short of breath' at the other end. The mark indicates the score and distance

- Do they have a stair lift installed?
- Do they have any rails indoors or by the outside steps?

Mobility is an intrinsic part of living and allows us to maintain a healthy and active lifestyle as well as independence. Lack of mobility can lead to total dependence on others, social isolation, frustration and depression. Questions to establish the problems the patient may experience while mobilising are important. Many patients will often require referral to a community physiotherapist for a mobility assessment for a suitable walking aid to help them regain their confidence and independence. Other patients may require a referral to social services for an assessment for installation of a stair lift, a ramp or outside rails to assist with their mobility. Many patients with severe COPD who are too breathless to walk any distance have invested in mobility scooters. This provides them with a new lease of life and independence to get to the shops to get their own shopping or to the post office/bank to withdraw some money. There are many different types on the market for patients to choose from.

5. Hygiene Needs and Dressing

Questions to ask:

- Are the patients independent with hygiene needs and dressing or do they need help?
- Are they able to shower or bath, and how often?
- Do they get breathless completing this task?
- Do they have to stop during the task, sit down or use their inhalers?
- How long does it take to complete this task?

General personal hygiene and grooming is a fundamental daily activity, not only to ensure cleanliness but also to keep warm/cool depending on the climate. Patients with moderate to severe breathlessness are likely to experience various degrees of breathlessness during this activity. If they are unable to bath or shower it is important to ascertain the reason why. It may be that with fitting some rails or a bath hoist they would find these activities more manageable. They may require a perch stool to wash or shave at the sink, as many patients are unable to stand for too long a period. Therefore referral to an occupational therapist would be relevant.

For many patients washing and dressing is a task that uses up a great deal of energy and may take them up to 45 minutes or more to complete this task, resting frequently and needing to use their inhalers. As health professionals it is essential not to just ask but also to observe a patient's cleanliness and whether he or she is managing to cope with this activity. Referral to social services for a home care package to help with this activity each morning and evening may be beneficial.

6. Nutrition

Questions to ask:

- Do they have a good appetite and eat regularly?
- Do they eat a well-balanced diet?
- Who does the shopping?
- Who prepares and cooks their meals? Do they have meals on wheels?
- How do they heat up their meals? (Some patients may only have a little tabletop cooker and stove ring or microwave.)
- Do they get breathless when eating?
- How much do they drink daily?
- Is their weight steady?
- What is their current weight (to calculate BMI)?

Eating and drinking, like breathing, is an essential activity to sustain life and keep healthy. Preparing and cooking meals involves a good part of each day. Many patients with COPD, particularly in its advanced stage, find eating very difficult, mainly due to their breathlessness, or have little appetite. If they live on their own they may be disinterested in eating alone and live on snacks rather than a balanced diet. Many elderly patients may not take adequate fluid to avoid visiting the toilet frequently and becoming extremely breathless following this activity. Not only is the amount of fluid intake per day important but also the type of fluid consumed. Many patients, particularly the elderly, drink tea but very little water. They should be encouraged to drink at least a couple of glasses a day as well as their cups of tea.

This particular activity is an area in which health professionals will need to invest a lot of time in providing patient advice and education surrounding nutritional issues. Referral to social services to arrange meals on wheels or advice from the community dietician may be appropriate.

7. Elimination

Questions to ask:

- Do they suffer from urinary stress incontinence or frequency?
- Are they ever incontinent?
- Do they have any problems passing water?
- Do they wake up at night to pass water?
- Are their bowels regular?
- Do they use laxatives on a regular basis?
- Are they prone to constipation?

Elimination, like eating and drinking, is a necessary bodily function and part of our everyday life. Many female patients with COPD suffer from urinary stress incontinence, particularly when coughing, sneezing or laughing – any activity that increases intra-abdominal pressure. Some patients may also suffer from urinary incontinence. Many of these patients suffer this embarrassing complaint silently and will never mention it to their GP. They spend huge amounts of their pension purchasing pads, which are not adequate to soak up the amount of urine they void. A majority of these patients may be on diuretic medication and as a result restrict their fluid intake to reduce the amount of urine they pass. Some patients may even avoid going out socially, particularly if worried about the availability of public toilets and are afraid of having an accident. Referral to the community incontinence service or district nurse for further assessment may help the patient tremendously and enhance their quality of life.

If constipation is a problem, advice with reference to a well-balanced diet with adequate fibre, fresh fruit and vegetables is important. Maintenance of an adequate fluid intake and exercise are also essential.

8. Sleeping

Questions to ask:

- Do they sleep well at night?
- How many hours do they sleep? Is this usual for them?
- What time do they usually go to bed and get up in the morning?
- Do they wake up during the night feeling breathless?
- Do they suffer from episodes of coughing at night?

- Do they need to use your inhaler, nebuliser or oxygen at any time during the night?
- How many pillows do they sleep with?
- If they do not sleep well, do they know the reason (i.e. pain due to arthritis)?

Sleep is an essential part of our lives. A good night's sleep enables us to rest and recharge our batteries. Sleeplessness or limited sleep will inevitably lead to tiredness and inability to cope. As individuals, the number of hour's sleep we require can vary. Some patients with a breathing problem may only get a couple of hours good-quality sleep a night. Therefore they will often complain of feeling tired and do not cope well with their condition. It is important to establish why they do not sleep. Night sedation is not advisable for patients with COPD due to the side effects, which may depress the respiratory centre.

9. Expressing Sexuality

This can be a rather uncomfortable topic to approach, not just for the patient but also for health professionals. However, for many patients it may be a subject they may wish to discuss or have anxieties about, but are too embarrassed to talk about. It is important to remember that although most patients with COPD may be older they may still be sexually active. Questions to ask:

- Do they have a sexually active relationship?
- Are there any issues or concerns that they wish to discuss?
- Are there any difficulties regarding sexual activity that are related to their breathing problem, which cause them or their partner concern?
- Does their breathlessness make them or their partner afraid to have sex?

10. Social Activities

Questions to ask:

- Do they go out at all? If so, is this with family, by car, taxi or by bus?
- If they do not go out, what prevents them from doing so?
- How many times a week/month do they go out?
- Where do they go?
- Do they belong to any social clubs or activity centres?

Such questions help to establish a little about their activities, their interests and the type of person they are as individuals. They also show whether they have a supportive family relationship. This type of information can be particularly useful to the health professional if the patient is not so well at home or is being discharged from hospital and may require some additional support at home for a short while.

11. Working and Playing

Questions to ask:

- Are they still working? If not, when did they retire/give up work and for what reason?
- Do they have any hobbies or interests in which they are able to partake?
- Do they do any physical activities such as walking or swimming?
- What do they do in their spare time?

These questions help to establish whether patients are still working and whether they have any difficulties or problems with their present employment which may require further advice. If patients are relatively young, it is interesting to find out, if they do not work, how they keep themselves occupied and what interests they have. Such nonmedical questions help to build up a picture about the patient and hopefully indicates that as a health professional you care about them as a person. This helps to establish a patient–health professional relationship where hopefully the patient develops a trusting relationship and feels able to discuss all issues related to his or her condition.

12. Dying

This activity is more to do with the journey as the patient's health declines and about preparing him or her and the carers in the actual process of dying. Many patients with end-stage COPD may have questions they would like to ask surrounding this subject if given the opportunity. It is a sensitive area and may be part of the assessment you may want to address at a further appointment, so as not to rush any issues the patient may have. As a health professional you are likely to pick up any vibes around this subject during the assessment from comments or remarks the patient or carer may make.

Concerns the patient may have may centre on issues such as:

- Fears on going to sleep and not waking up
- Feeling of impending death during an exacerbation, particularly when very breathless or during a severe coughing bout
- Will they die struggling for breath or be in pain?
- Will their death be like drowning?
- Concerns around issues of resuscitation if admitted to hospital with respiratory failure

- Issues regarding living wills
- Their wish to die at home if their condition deteriorates

It may not just be the patient that has concerns about dying, but also the carers, particularly if elderly and dependent on the patient. The fear of how they will cope once the loved one has gone can be a worrying time. After the event, it can bring intense loneliness and difficulties managing on their own. It is not unusual that within a year of losing a wife or husband the spouse also dies, usually of a broken heart (Roper, Logan and Tierney, 2001).

RESPIRATORY EXAMINATION OF THE PATIENT

General Examination – First Impressions

The examination starts when the patient is first met either in the clinic or at home. Initial impressions are important to assist in developing a clinical picture and confirming a diagnosis. The following points should be observed:

- How breathless does the patient appear on walking into the room or answering the door?
- Is the patient able to talk following exertion, or does he or she need to rest before continuing with the conversation?
- Does the patient appear distressed by breathlessness?
- How is the patient's colour? Does he or she appear cyanosed, particularly around the lips, pale or flushed?
- Is the patient coughing?
- Does the patient appear wheezy?
- How is the patient breathing? Is the breathing through pursed lips? Is the breathing rapid, shallow or deep? Is the patient using accessory muscles to breathe (e.g. scalenes, sternocleidomastoids), signifying some element of respiratory difficulty?

After completing an assessment of the patient's symptoms, medical history and medication prescribed, a physical examination will assist the health professional in acquiring further information about the patient and his or her general health.

For a physical examination it is important to expose the patient to the waist. Ensure that there is adequate light, the room is warm and the patient is well sat up and comfortable. If examining the patient in the home, this examination can either take place with the patient in a chair or positioned on the bed, depending on the circumstances and the condition of the patient.

It is advisable for the health professional to develop a systematic approach to examining the patient to perform a thorough and professional examination. A suggested systematic approach to examination is as follows.

OBSERVATIONS

Examine both hands for the following:

- Examination of the fingers may reveal tar staining from tobacco.
- Finger clubbing is not a specific feature of COPD but may alert the clinician to other underlying lung disease such as cancer (Table 3.4). It can be identified by the increased sponginess of the nail bed, loss of acute angle between the nail and nail bed, increased nail curvature and increased bulk of the soft tissue over the terminal phalanges. With advanced finger clubbing the whole tip of the finger becomes rounded like a club (Figure 3.1). Finger

Table 3.4. Causes of finger clubbing

Respiratory
Bronchiectais
Bronchial carcinoma
Cystic fibrosis
Fibrosing alveolitis
Asbestosis
Lung abscess
Empyema
Mesothelioma
Cardiac
Cyanotic congenital heart disease
Infective endocarditis
Other
Idiopathic/hereditary
Ulcerative colitis
Crohn's disease
Cirrhosis of the liver

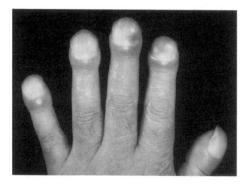

Figure 3.1. A slide showing finger clubbing. By courtesy of Dr C.R. McGavin, Derriford Hospital, Plymouth

clubbing may occasionally be hereditary in otherwise normal subjects. However, the mechanism of finger clubbing is not fully understood. It may occur rapidly, but usually its onset is gradual.

- In peripheral cyanosis the colour of the fingers and nail beds may be blue and reflect central cyanosis if the fingers are warm. If cold this may reflect poor peripheral perfusion, as seen in Raynaud's phenomenon or peripheral vascular disease.
- Carbon dioxide retention can be found in severe COPD. Clinically this can be detected by requesting the patient to hold their hands outstretched. An irregular flapping tremor will be noted and the hands will feel strikingly warm and the pulses bounding.

Record observations of the following:

- Document the patient's temperature.
- Check the pulse and note the rate and rhythm.
- Record the blood pressure.
- Count the respiratory rate, noting the rate, breathing pattern, use of any accessory muscles of breathing (e.g. scalenes, sternocleidomastoids) or pursed lip breathing. Tachypnea with rapid shallow breathing, with a prolonged expiratory phase, is an important clinical sign of COPD, particularly in emphysema.

Head and neck observations include:

- Check the eyes for evidence of anaemia, which may indicate a cause of breathlessness.
- Observe the colour of the tongue for evidence of central cyanosis, which will be seen to be bluish (except in Black and Asian nationalities).
- Check under the chin around the supraclavicular area and cervical nodes for lymphadenopathy.
- Check that the trachea is central. The distance between the suprasternal notch and the cricoid cartilage is normally 3–4 fingers in an adult. Deviation of the trachea suggests another chest disease other than COPD.
- Observe for evidence of jugular venous pressure (JVP), which may be raised in cor pulmonale (right-sided heart failure) associated with lung disease. The patient should be positioned preferably at a 30° angle and the patient's head turned to the side to expose the area of the carotid artery. A good light is essential to see clearly whether it is elevated. Pressures measured more than 3–4 cm above the sternal angle is considered elevated.

Peripheral oedema:

• Peripheral oedema is commonly evident in patients with severe COPD and cor pulmonale. The degree of ankle oedema should be noted and whether the oedema is pitting.

Physical Examination of the Chest

Though a general physical examination is an integral part of assessing the patient, it must be remembered that a diagnosis cannot be made purely on an examination alone. Any findings must be used in conjunction with symptoms, a chest X-ray and spirometry. The process followed in the physical respiratory examination is:

• Inspection
• Palpation
• Percussion
• Auscultation

INSPECTION OF THE CHEST WALL – FRONT

1. Observe the size and shape of the chest wall for any abnormalities particularly relevant to patients with chronic lung disease, such as a barrel chest demonstrating lung hyperinflation or pectus excavatum (funnel chest) where the sternum is depressed. In pectus carinatum (pigeon chest), the sternum and costal cartilages project outwards. Note any scars from previous cardiac or thoracic surgery.
2. Systematically palpate the chest wall for tenderness, masses or crepitus.
3. Note the rate, depth and regularity of the breathing. Check if the chest expands equally each side of the chest. This is conducted by placing both hands on the chest wall and as the patient takes a deep breath in, watch for divergence of thumbs as the chest wall expands – both sides of the chest should expand equally (Figure 3.2). Poor chest expansion in patients with COPD is a significant sign of hyperinflation.
4. Palpate the cardiac apex, which is normally located at, or medial to, the midclavicular line in the fourth to fifth interspace.
5. Percussion of the chest is a technique used to determine differences in percussion note over the lung field and takes some practice to perfect. This procedure is conducted (if right-handed) by placing the fingers of the left hand on the chest with the fingers separated and striking the middle finger with the terminal phalynx using the middle finger of the right hand briskly. The striking movement should be a flick of the wrist and the striking finger should be at right angles to the other finger. As well as noting the sound of the percussion, vibration may be felt on the

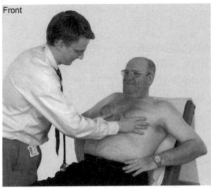
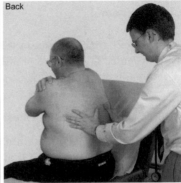

Figure 3.2. Demonstrating the technique to check chest expansion

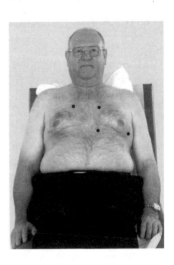

Figure 3.3. Indicating the position of the stethoscope to auscultate heart sounds

chest wall. The percussion note is resonant over aerated lung and hyper-
resonant when emphysema or bullae are present. Resonance is decreased
moderately in consolidation and fibrosis. If pleural fluid is present a stony
dullness will be noted.

6. Carry out auscultation of the heart (using the bell of the stethoscope) in
the four auscultatory areas of the chest, listening to the first and second
heart sounds – S1 and S2 (lub/dub) – for irregularities and murmurs
(Figure 3.3):

- Aortic (second right interspace)
- Pulmonary (second left interspace)
- Tricuspid (sternal border)
- Mitral (at apex)

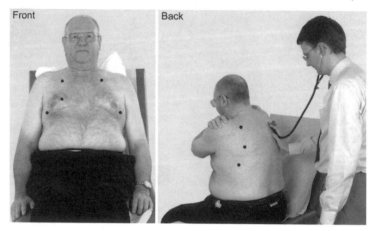

Figure 3.4. Indicating the position of the stethoscope to auscultate breath sounds

7. Carry out auscultation of the lungs. It is important to listen to the lungs in a systematic pattern comparing sides. Patients with COPD often have reduced breath sounds, but this finding is not sufficiently characteristic to confirm a diagnosis. Ask the patient to take deep breaths through the mouth and, starting at the apices and using the diaphragm of the stethoscope, listen to the anterior fields in a methodical sequence over the chest (Figure 3.4, left).

INSPECTION OF THE SPINE AND BACK

8. Ask the patient to lean forward and observe the spine for any deformities such as kyphosis (forward curvature of the spine) or scoliosis (lateral curvature of the spine). Also note any scars that may relate to previous thoracic surgery.
9. Systematically palpate the back for tenderness, masses or crepitus.
10. To auscultate the back of the chest, ask the patient to cross their arms and place their hands on the top of their shoulders (Figure 3.4, right). This manoeuvre assists listening to the chest by moving the shoulder blades from the lung fields. Again it is important to listen to the lungs in a systematic pattern, comparing sides. Ask the patient to take deep breaths through the mouth, which forces a greater volume of air in the lungs, increasing the duration, intensity and ability to detect any abnormal breath sounds. Starting at the apices and using the diaphragm of the stethoscope, listen to the posterior fields in a methodical sequence over the chest. First start with the upper aspect of the posterior fields on both sides and by repeating the process listen in four places on each side of the chest. If anything abnormal is heard, then listen in more places. At least

two breath cycles should be heard to detect any abnormal breath sounds in each area. Prior knowledge of which lobe of the lung is heard best in each region is relevant in trying to make an accurate diagnosis: lower lobes occupy the lower three-quarters of the posterior fields; the right middle lobe is heard in the right axilla and the lingula in the left axilla.

BREATH SOUNDS

Vesicular breath sounds are normal usually heard over normal lungs on inspiration and the first part of expiration. Reduction in vesicular breath sounds may be detected in asthma and emphysema. Auscultation of patients with severe, stable emphysema will produce very little sound. Additional sounds that may be detected are:

- Bronchial breathing is when the breath sounds become harsh and high pitched due to enhanced transmission of sound through abnormal lung, such as in areas of consolidation.
- Wheezes are musical sounds, which are produced during expiration when air is forced through airways narrowed by bronchoconstriction or secretions. On auscultation a wheeze is relatively high pitched with a hissing or shrill quality. In asthma, chronic bronchitis and emphysema multiple polyphonic wheezes may be heard on expiration, usually throughout the lungs. Occasionally, focal wheezing can occur when airway narrowing is restricted to a single area, as might occur with an obstructing tumour or consolidation due to pneumonia.
- Crackles (crepitations or rales) are short explosive sounds similar to that produced by rubbing strands of hair together close to the ear. These represent abrupt opening of collapsed small airways during inspiration and are associated with processes that cause fluid to accumulate within the alveolar and interstitial spaces. It is important to note whether the crackles are localised to one area such as in pneumonia. However, in pulmonary oedema both lung bases would be equally affected.
- Pleural rub is the sound produced when two layers of abnormal pleura move over one another in a jerky motion, generating a creaking sound similar to that produced by bending stiff leather. Rubs are usually heard on both inspiration and expiration and are associated with pleural inflammation.

11. To assist with diagnosis and confirmation of findings it may be useful to conduct a procedure known as vocal resonance. This is done by placing the stethoscope on the chest and requesting the patient to say 'ninety-nine'. Normally the sound produced is 'fuzzy'. In areas of consolidation the sound is increased, and decreased if there is air, fluid or pleural thickening between the lung and the chest wall. In some cases, even when

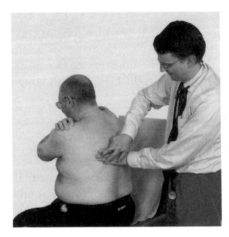

Figure 3.5. Demonstrating the technique for percussion of the back of the chest

patients whisper, the sound is still clearly heard over the affected lung (whispering pectoriloquy).

12. Percussion of the back of the chest following auscultation again assists to confirm findings (Figure 3.5). When percussing the chest, comparison should be made between identical areas on both sides in an attempt to detect differences in percussion notes. The percussion note is resonant over aerated lung and hyper-resonant when emphysema or bullae are present. Resonance is decreased moderately in consolidation and fibrosis. If pleural fluid is present a stony dullness will be noted.

SUMMARY

COPD is a condition with a gradual onset that causes breathlessness on exertion, chronic cough with or without production of sputum, occasional wheeze and frequent infective exacerbations. It is usually a condition that follows many decades of cigarette smoking and/or exposure to other risk factors such as occupational or environmental factors. In establishing an accurate diagnosis it is essential to obtain a thorough history and presenting symptoms as well as the impact this has on the patient's daily activities of living. The findings following a physical examination of the chest will assist in forming a diagnosis in conjunction with other investigations, as described in Chapter 4.

Chapter 4

Investigations to Diagnose COPD

INTRODUCTION

Investigations are essential to confirm a diagnosis of COPD in addition to obtaining a good history and a thorough examination. Any patient over the age of 35 years of age presenting with a history of smoking (or an ex-smoker) and symptoms of breathlessness, such as a cough with sputum production, should be further investigated. Respiratory diagnostic investigations include:

- Lung function testing
- Chest X-ray
- Computerised tomography scan
- Sputum culture
- Pulse oximetry
- Arterial blood gas analysis

LUNG FUNCTION TESTING

Once COPD is suspected on clinical grounds, the diagnosis and degree of airflow obstruction is best assessed by spirometry. Spirometry is the gold standard for accurately measuring the airflow obstruction in patients with COPD. Peak expiratory flow (PEF) rates are not of particular value in the diagnosis of COPD, unlike asthma, as airflow is only measured from the upper large airways. Also PEF does not differentiate between restrictive and obstructive airways disease, and is therefore not diagnostic with regards to COPD.

WHAT IS SPIROMETRY?

'Spiro' is the Greek word for 'breathing'. Therefore spirometry is defined as the measurement of breathing. The first spirometer was developed in 1846 by Hutchinson (Johns and Pierce, 2003). Spirometry is a simple test to measure the maximum volume of air a person can exhale, and the time taken to do so. Since the implementation of the COPD guidelines (National Collaborating Centre for Chronic Conditions, 2004) and the new General Medical Services (GMS) contracts, many practice nurses are now performing spirometry. However, the usefulness of spirometry measurements relies upon the accuracy of the spirometer, care and maintenance of the equipment, interpretation of results, as well as the competence of the person performing the test.

TYPES OF SPIROMETERS

There are many devices on the market with costs varying from £300 to over £3000. Whichever type of spirometer is used, it is preferable that a visible volume–time graph is available to check the curve produced by the patient.

Volume Displacement Spirometers

A dry wedge bellows such as the Vitalograph 2150 (Figure 4.1) consists of a set of bellows mounted in a box. As the patient blows into the bellows through a connecting tube, these expand, which allows a stylus pen on the top of the machine to provide a tracing on a graph. The time on the chart/graph trace is typically 6 or 12 seconds, although it is important to note that the subject should continue to exhale even if the end is reached in order to record all of the volume fully.

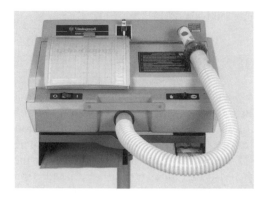

Figure 4.1. Vitalograph spirometer

Flow-Sensing Spirometers

Pneumotachograph models such as the Vitalograph 2120 and Alpha 111 have an internal electronic transducer, which measures the pressure difference before and after an obstruction in the flow head as the patient blows. A pressure transducer is used to measure the flow rate from which the volume is derived:

$$\text{Flow} = \frac{\text{pressure difference}}{\text{resistance}}$$

The digital turbine/rotary vane includes models such as the MicroMedical MicroLoop and MicroLab (Figure 4.2). As the patient blows into the spirometer an internal vane rotates and two light-emitting diodes count the number of rotations. The number of rotations with time directly measures the flow rate from which the volume is then derived.

SPIROMETRY MEASUREMENTS USED TO DIAGNOSE COPD

Spirometry is an essential tool in the diagnosis of COPD because it can differentiate between restrictive and obstructive disease. It may also be used as a screening tool in smokers (with a smoking history greater than 10 years) to detect early changes before any significant symptoms are evident. It is the most widely used lung function test as it can:

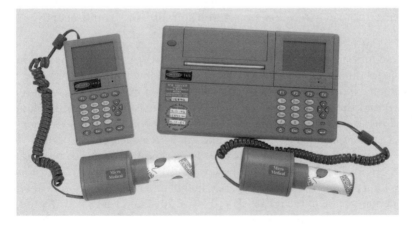

Figure 4.2. MicroMedical MicroLoop and MicroLab spirometers

- Provide an accurate diagnosis
- Indicate the severity of the disease
- Ensure appropriate drug management
- Objectively assess effects of drugs prescribed
- Assess the progression of the disease based on objective measurements
- Provide information about the prognosis
- Is reasonably quick, cheap and portable

Patterns of airflow are determined by the following measurements:

- FEV_1 (forced expired volume in one second) is the volume of air exhaled in the first second of forced expiration after maximal inspiration.
- FVC (forced vital capacity) is the maximum volume of air that can be forcibly exhaled from maximum inhalation (total lung capacity) to maximum exhalation (residual volume) measured against time.
- FEV_1/FVC is the ratio of FEV_1 to FVC expressed as a percentage, which is calculated as follows:

$$\frac{FEV_1}{FVC} \times 100 = FEV_1/FVC \text{ ratio}$$

- RVC (relaxed vital capacity) is a nonforced expiration measurement, which is often greater than the FVC in patients with COPD. The patients blow out at their own pace after maximal inhalation with a nose clip in place. In patients with emphysema where airways collapse during a forced blow, it may give a more accurate measurement. Ideally the largest volume recorded should be used as a vital capacity (VC) in the FEV_1/VC ratio.
- PEF (peak expiratory flow) is the maximum flow that a patient can achieve during a forced expiration from full inspiration in 10 milliseconds.

These measurements, with the exception of RVC, are made by asking the patient to inhale to maximum capacity and blow out hard and fast until maximum expiration is reached. The volume of air expelled in the first second (FEV_1) and the total volume (FVC, RVC) is measured. When divided, this provides the proportion exhaled in the first second. Spirometry measures FEV_1 that is reproducible, objective and allows a measurement of the severity of the disease to be categorised. COPD is classified as mild, moderate or severe (Table 4.1), depending on the level of FEV_1 compared to the reference values for a person of a similar age, sex, height and race. A diagnosis of airflow obstruction can be made if the FEV_1/FVC < 70% and FEV_1 < 80% predicted (National Collaborating Centre for Chronic Conditions, 2004). For example:

Table 4.1. Classification of COPD. Taken from National Collaborating Centre for Chronic Conditions (2004)

Category	Symptoms	Signs
Mild (FEV$_1$ 50–80% predicted)	Smokers cough; minimal breathlessness	None
Moderate (FEV$_1$ 30–49% predicted)	Breathlessness and/or wheeze; cough and/or sputum	Few signs
Severe (FEV$_1$ <30% predicted)	Breathlessness on minimal exertion; cough, wheeze	Hyperinflation; hypoxia; peripheral oedema

Patient: Age: 62 years old
       Sex: female
       Height: 160 cm

$$\text{FEV}_1 \quad \frac{\text{Reading} \quad 0.86}{\text{Predicted value} \quad 2.00} \times 100\% = 43\% \text{ of normal predicted}$$

$$\text{FVC} \quad \frac{\text{Reading} \quad 1.96}{\text{Predicted value} \quad 2.40} \times 100\% = 82\% \text{ of normal predicted}$$

$$\text{FEV}_1/\text{FVC} \quad \frac{\text{Reading} \quad 0.86}{\text{Reading} \quad 1.96} \times 100\% = 44\%$$

Interpretation

The patient has moderate airflow obstruction as FEV$_1$ is between 30 and 50% of the predicted normal, and FEV$_1$/FVC is < 70%.

COMPLICATIONS AND CONTRAINDICATIONS TO PERFORMING SPIROMETRY

Spirometry is a relatively safe and noninvasive procedure. However, it does require maximal effort and cooperation from the patient. For some patients, it may cause breathlessness, cough and light-headedness. For a small minority of patients it may even induce a degree of bronchospasm. There are a number of clinical circumstances where spirometry is not advisable because the increased intrathoracic pressure may affect other parts of the body. These include the following:

- Recent eye surgery
- Recent thoracic, abdominal surgery or aneurysm

- Pneumothorax
- Chest or abdominal pain
- Haemoptysis
- Unstable cardiac function or recent myocardial infarction
- Vomiting and diarrhoea

PREPARATION OF THE PATIENT FOR SPIROMETRY

Prior to the test, patients need to be adequately prepared. Patients should have been clinically stable for 4–6 weeks to make an accurate diagnosis of COPD. Ideally the patient should avoid the following before attempting spirometry (Association of Respiratory Technicians and Physiologists/British Thoracic Society, 1994):

- Smoking for 24 hours
- Drinking alcohol for at least 4 hours
- Eating a large meal at least 2 hours before the test
- Taking short-acting bronchodilators for 6 hours
- Taking long-acting beta-2-agonist inhalers for 12 hours
- Taking any slow-release medications that affect respiratory function and theophylline-based drugs for 24 hours
- Vigorous exercise for at least 30 minutes
- Wearing any tight clothing

Note that patients should be encouraged to empty their bladders prior to testing.

PROCEDURE FOR SPIROMETRY

- The patient's age, height (without shoes), sex and ethnicity should be documented.
- A full explanation of what the procedure involves should be provided and demonstrated.
- The patient should be seated in an upright position. This is as a precaution in case the patient feels light-headed or dizzy, and to standardise the results.
- The patient should be instructed to take a full inspiration through the mouth and to place the mouthpiece in the mouth, ensuring the lips and teeth are securely around the mouthpiece to form a tight seal.
- The patient is instructed to blow out, forcibly, as hard and as fast as possible, until there is nothing left to expel. Patients will require some encourage-

ment to keep blowing to provide a complete blow. The FVC should take at least 6 seconds, although for some patients with severe COPD this may take up to 15 seconds.

- A minimum of three attempts and a maximum of eight attempts should be made at any one time. At least two readings of FEV_1 within at least 100 ml or 5% of each other are recorded to ensure good reproducibility. The expiratory volume/time traces should be smooth, convex upwards and with no irregularities in the curve due to coughing or reduced effort.

COMMON REASONS FOR INCONSISTENT SPIROMETRY RESULTS

The most common reason for inconsistent results is patient technique. During the procedure the patient should be observed to detect any errors and the tracing on the graph examined (Figure 4.3). Common problems include:

- Submaximal effort from the patient during the procedure
- Not full inspiration
- Lips not tight around the mouthpiece, causing leakage
- Additional breath during the procedure
- A slow start to the forced exhalation
- Coughing during exhalation
- Early termination of the procedure before complete exhalation

INTERPRETING THE RESULTS OF SPIROMETRY

The best of the three consistent spirometry readings is selected. Most spirometers will calculate the predicted normal values and the results in percentages once the patient's details of sex, age and height have been entered (Figure 4.4). Exceptions to this are the wedge bellow device, which will require reading of the graph paper, and the percentage of the predicted normal values for the patient can be calculated by referring to various tables available. The most relevant tables used in the UK are those published by the European Community for Steel and Coal (Quanjer *et al.*, 1993).

Spirometry results are vital to determine the patient's lung function into one of four different disease patterns or classifications:

- Normal
- Obstructive
- Restrictive
- Mixed

Quality Assurance

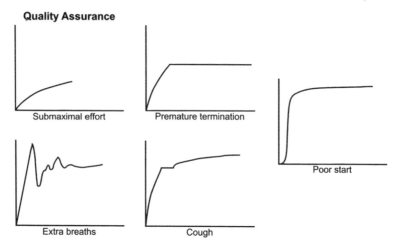

Submaximal effort · Premature termination · Poor start · Extra breaths · Cough

Figure 4.3. Demonstrating common problems in performing spirometry and producing poor results. Reproduced by permission of Vitalograph

Predicted normal values

These values apply to Caucasians. Reduce values by 7% for Asians and by 13% for Afro-Caribbeans.

Male		5'3" 160cm	5'5" 165cm	5'7" 170cm	5'9" 175cm	5'11" 180cm	6'1" 185cm	6'3" 190cm
38-41 years	FVC	3.81	4.10	4.39	4.67	4.96	5.25	5.54
	FEV₁	3.20	3.42	3.63	3.85	4.06	4.28	4.49
42-45 years	FVC	3.71	3.99	4.28	4.57	4.86	5.15	5.43
	FEV₁	3.09	3.30	3.52	3.73	3.95	4.16	4.38
46-49 years	FVC	3.60	3.89	4.18	4.47	4.75	5.04	5.33
	FEV₁	2.97	3.18	3.40	3.61	3.83	4.04	4.26
50-53 years	FVC	3.50	3.79	4.07	4.36	4.65	4.94	5.23
	FEV₁	2.85	3.07	3.28	3.50	3.71	3.93	4.14
54-57 years	FVC	3.39	3.68	3.97	4.26	4.55	4.83	5.12
	FEV₁	2.74	2.95	3.17	3.38	3.60	3.81	4.03
58-61 years	FVC	3.29	3.58	3.87	4.15	4.44	4.73	5.02
	FEV₁	2.62	2.84	3.05	3.27	3.48	3.70	3.91
62-65 years	FVC	3.19	3.47	3.76	4.05	4.34	4.63	4.91
	FEV₁	2.51	2.72	2.94	3.15	3.37	3.58	3.80
66-69 years	FVC	3.08	3.37	3.66	3.95	4.23	4.52	4.81
	FEV₁	2.39	2.60	2.82	3.03	3.25	3.46	3.68

For men over 70 years, predicted values are less well established but can be calculated from the equations below (height in cms; age in years):
$FVC = (0.0576 \times height) - (0.026 \times age) - 4.34$ (SD: ± 0.61 litres)
$FEV_1 = (0.043 \times height) - (0.029 \times age) - 2.49$ (SD: ± 0.51 litres)

Female		4'11" 150cm	5'1" 155cm	5'3" 160cm	5'5" 165cm	5'7" 170cm	5'9" 175cm	5'11" 180cm
38-41 years	FVC	2.69	2.91	3.13	3.35	3.58	3.80	4.02
	FEV₁	2.30	2.50	2.70	2.89	3.09	3.29	3.49
42-45 years	FVC	2.59	2.81	3.03	3.25	3.47	3.69	3.91
	FEV₁	2.20	2.40	2.60	2.79	2.99	3.19	3.39
46-49 years	FVC	2.48	2.70	2.92	3.15	3.37	3.59	3.81
	FEV₁	2.10	2.30	2.50	2.69	2.89	3.09	3.29
50-53 years	FVC	2.38	2.60	2.82	3.04	3.26	3.48	3.71
	FEV₁	2.00	2.20	2.40	2.59	2.79	2.99	3.19
54-57 years	FVC	2.27	2.49	2.72	2.94	3.16	3.38	3.60
	FEV₁	1.90	2.10	2.30	2.49	2.69	2.89	3.09
58-61 years	FVC	2.17	2.39	2.61	2.83	3.06	3.28	3.50
	FEV₁	1.80	2.00	2.20	2.39	2.59	2.79	2.99
62-65 years	FVC	2.07	2.29	2.51	2.73	2.95	3.17	3.39
	FEV₁	1.70	1.90	2.10	2.29	2.49	2.69	2.89
66-69 years	FVC	1.96	2.18	2.40	2.63	2.85	3.07	3.29
	FEV₁	1.60	1.80	2.00	2.19	2.39	2.59	2.79

For women over 70 years, predicted values are less well established but can be calculated from the equations below (height in cms; age in years):
$FVC = (0.0443 \times height) - (0.026 \times age) - 2.89$ (SD: ± 0.43 litres)
$FEV_1 = (0.0395 \times height) - (0.025 \times age) - 2.60$ (SD: ± 0.36 litres)

BTS COPD Consortium; Spirometry in practice: A practical guide to using spirometry in primary care September 2000.

SPI/SPV 952
Date of preparation: March 2005

Figure 4.4. Predicted values for FEV₁ and FVC in men and women. Reproduced by permission of Boehringer Ingelheim

Most electronic spirometers are able to produce two types of graphs, the flow/volume loop and the volume/time curve. The flow/volume loop measures flow on the *y* axis (in litres per second or litres per minute) and volume (in litres) on the *x* axis (Figure 4.5(a)). The volume/time curve measures the volume in litres on the vertical axis (*y*) and time in seconds on the horizontal axis (*x*). It is from this curve that the measurements for FEV_1 and FVC are calculated (Figure 4.5(b)).

The significance of the flow/volume curve is that it can give an insight into what is happening in the smaller airways of the lungs. Figures 4.6 and 4.7 give examples of mild and moderate airflow obstructions. In severe emphysema the flow/volume curve often resembles a church steeple due to the rapid collapse of the airways and air trapping during forced expiration as a result of loss of elastic tissue support (Figure 4.8).

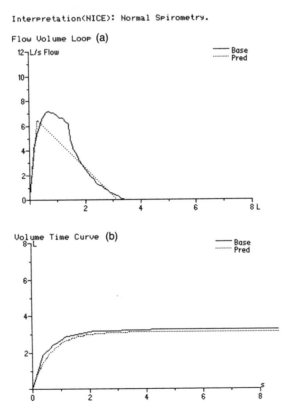

Figure 4.5. Normal (a) flow/volume loop and (b) volume/time curve

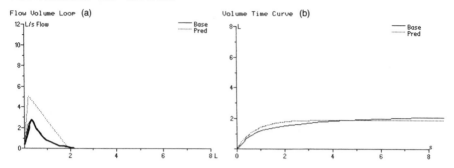

Figure 4.6. Mild obstruction demonstrated

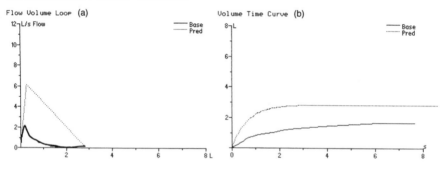

Figure 4.7. Moderate obstruction demonstrated

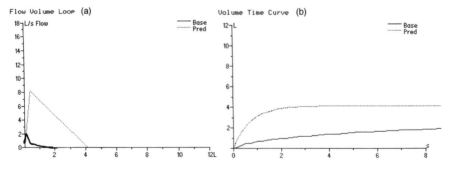

Figure 4.8. Severe obstruction demonstrated

Normal Spirometry

When the airways and lung tissue are normal, most of the air, 70–85%, will be expelled from the lungs in the first second (FEV_1) (Figure 4.9):

- FEV_1 > 80% predicted normal
- FVC > 80% predicted normal
- FEV_1/FVC ratio > 70%

For example:
$$FEV_1 = 2.59 \text{ litres and FVC} = 3.04 \text{ litres}$$

$$FEV_1/FVC \text{ ratio} = \frac{2.59}{3.04} \times 100 = 79\%, \text{ indicating normal spirometry}$$

Obstructive Pattern

This refers to any disease that may affect the calibre of the airways due to excessive mucous production, inflammation, bronchoconstriction and loss of lung recoil. As a result, the rate at which the air can be exhaled is reduced, thereby reducing the FEV_1. A classic obstructive pattern shows reduced flow rates and normal lung volumes within the FVC. Diseases that may cause an obstructive pattern are COPD, asthma, bronchiectasis and cystic fibrosis (Figure 4.10):

- FEV_1 – reduced (< 80% predicted normal)
- FVC – normal or reduced
- FEV_1/FVC ratio – reduced

For example:
$$FEV_1 = 1.19 \text{ litres and FVC} = 2.56 \text{ litres}$$

$$FEV_1/FVC \text{ ratio} = \frac{1.19}{2.56} \times 100 = 46\%, \text{ indicating a moderate obstructive pattern}$$

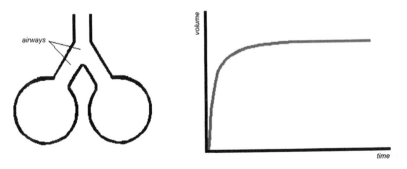

Figure 4.9. Representation of normal lungs and airways with the corresponding spirogram. Reproduced by permission of Vitalograph

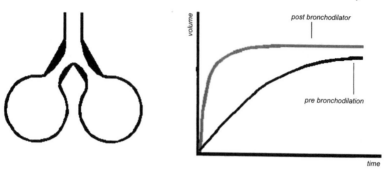

Figure 4.10. Representation of the lungs and airways with the corresponding spirogram showing a pattern of airways obstruction. Reproduced by permission of Vitalograph

Restrictive Pattern

A restrictive pattern is one that affects the lung tissue as a result of fibrosis or scarring, or an inability of the lungs to expand due to a physical deformity of the chest wall or muscular weakness. The airways are normal in restrictive disease so the flow of air is not restricted, but the lung volume is reduced. Therefore the restrictive pattern presents as reduced volumes with normal flow rates (Figure 4.11). Conditions that may produce a restrictive pattern are fibrosing alveolitis, asbestosis, kyphoscoliosis, pleural effusion or obesity:

- FEV_1 – reduced
- FVC – reduced
- FEV_1/FVC ratio – normal or increased

For example:

$$FEV_1 = 1.70 \text{ litres and FVC} = 1.95 \text{ litres}$$

$$FEV_1/FVC \text{ ratio} = \frac{1.70}{1.95} \times 100 = 87\%, \text{ indicating a restrictive pattern}$$

Mixed Pattern

A mixed pattern is a disease that affects both the airways and the lung tissue and therefore shows features of obstructive and restrictive disease (Figure 4.12). Conditions that may produce a combined pattern are severe COPD, advanced bronchiectais and cystic fibrosis:

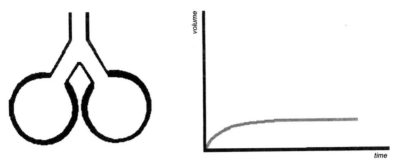

Figure 4.11. Representation of the lungs and airways with the corresponding spirogram showing a pattern of airways restriction. Reproduced by permission of Vitalograph

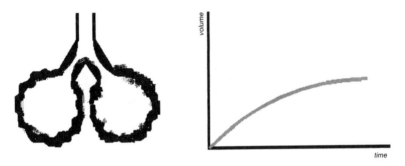

Figure 4.12. Representation of the lungs and airways with the corresponding spirogram showing a pattern of mixed airways disease. Reproduced by permission of Vitalograph

- FEV_1 – reduced
- FVC – reduced or normal
- FEV_1/FVC ratio – reduced

For example:

$$FEV_1 = 1.16 \text{ litres and FVC} = 2.24 \text{ litres}$$

$$FEV_1/FVC \text{ ratio} = \frac{1.16}{2.24} \times 100 = 52\%, \text{indicating a mixed pattern}$$

REVERSIBILITY TESTING

While spirometry remains essential for confirming the diagnosis of airflow obstruction, the NICE COPD guidelines (National Collaborating Centre for Chronic Conditions, 2004) no longer recommend that reversibility testing be carried out on all patients. It is felt that COPD or asthma can usually be determined on clinical grounds (Table 4.2). This argument is based on several clinical studies, which have shown that routine reversibility testing may be unhelpful or misleading, since reversibility tests performed on the same patient on different occasions give inconsistent and variable results and are therefore not reproducible. Over-reliance could potentially be placed on a single reversibility result, leading to an inaccurate diagnosis. However, these recommendations conflict with the new GP GMS contract, which stipulates that spirometry with reversibility testing is required. At present this discrepancy is under review with the Department of Health.

OTHER USEFUL INVESTIGATIONS

Chest X-Ray

A chest X-ray is seldom diagnostic in the early stages of COPD but it may be valuable in excluding an alternative diagnosis such as bronchial carcinoma. A normal chest X-ray will show the following (Figure 4.13):

- Shape and size of the heart
- Lung fields and pleura
- Rib cage
- Diaphragm
- Bony structures
- Soft tissue outline of the breasts

Table 4.2. Clinical features differentiating COPD and asthma. Taken from National Collaborating Centre for Chronic Conditions (2004)

	COPD	Asthma
Smoker or ex-smoker	Nearly all	Possible
Symptoms under age 35	Rare	Common
Chronic productive cough	Common	Uncommon
Breathlessness	Persistent and progressive	Variable
Night-time waking with breathlessness and/or wheeze	Uncommon	Common
Significant diurnal or day-to-day variability of symptoms	Uncommon	Common

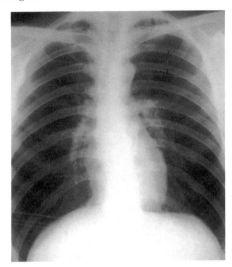

Figure 4.13. Normal chest X-ray. By courtesy of Dr C.R. McGavin, Derriford Hospital, Plymouth

Radiological changes associated with COPD are large lungs due to air trapping, which will extend to the seventh or eighth rib anteriorly. The diaphragm may appear flat or scallop shaped, instead of concave upwards, due to hyperexpansion of the lungs. There may also be evidence of fewer blood vessels visible peripherally, especially in the upper and middle zones (Figure 4.14). In patients with an exacerbation or those who are not responding to treatment, a plain chest X-ray is useful in excluding lobar pneumonia or pneumothorax.

Computerised Tomography Scan

The image display of computerised tomography (CT) is different to the image projected by a chest X-ray (Figure 4.15). It is much more sensitive, which produces cross-sectional images of the CT and can accurately locate lesions more readily than from a chest X-ray. A computerised tomography scan is not routinely conducted for COPD unless either there is doubt about the diagnosis or if a surgical procedure such as bullectomy or lung volume reduction is being considered.

Haematology

Identification of anaemia in the management of patients with COPD is useful, as this may be a cause of breathlessness. Polycythaemia can develop in patients

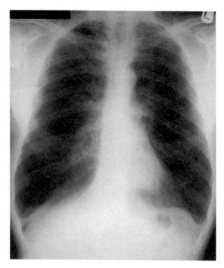

Figure 4.14. Chest X-ray showing COPD. Both lungs appear blacker and larger in volume. Hemidiaphragms are flattened

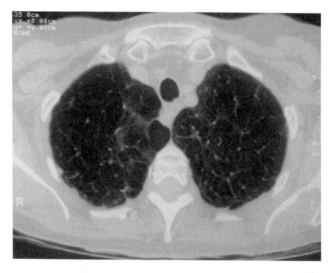

Figure 4.15. CT showing emphysema

with chronic hypoxaemia. Venesection should be considered if the packed cell volume (PCV) is greater than 60% in men and 55% in women, although the evidence for its benefits to reduce the above risks is rather limited (Halpin, 2003).

The white cell count may be elevated during an infective exacerbation, particularly if infection is not confined to the bronchi but has spread to the lung parenchyma, as in pneumonia (Bourke, 2003). It is also important to assess for any electrolyte disturbance (sodium and potassium levels) in patients with acute exacerbations requiring frequent nebulised bronchodilator drugs.

Electrocardiogram

An electrocardiogram (ECG) is useful for detecting ischaemic heart disease and arrhythmias. Patients with cor pulmonale may show features of right ventricular hypertrophy (right axis deviation, dominant R wave in V_1).

Sputum Culture

Routine culture of nonpurulent sputum is of no value in the management or evaluation of patients with COPD (Barnes, 1999). Sputum is frequently colonised in this group of patients with bacteria such as *Haemophilus influenzae*, whose identification without other symptoms is not an indication for antibiotic therapy. However, sputum culture may be useful in confirming what organisms are present and in detecting resistance to antibiotics.

Alpha-1 Antitrypsin Deficiency Screening

A rare risk factor for COPD is an inherited deficiency of alpha-1 antitrypsin. This enzyme prevents the destruction of proteolytic enzymes in the lung. In those patients who develop emphysema between the ages of 20 and 40 years or who have a strong family history of the disease, alpha-1 antitrypsin should be measured. A serum concentration of alpha-1 antitrypsin below 15–20% of the normal value is highly suggestive of homozygous alpha-1 antitrypsin deficiency, and further testing should be pursued.

Pulse Oximetry

Measuring oxygen saturations using a pulse oximeter is a useful and noninvasive procedure. Pulse oximetry can be used to assess the patient's oxygen levels at rest and post-exertion when stable and during an exacerbation.

The pulse oximeter measures the amount of oxygen that is combined with haemoglobin. This is referred to as oxygen saturation (SaO_2) and is expressed as a percentage. In healthy adults the normal range is greater than 95% for air. Pulse oximeters are compact and portable, which provide a continuous digital display of (Figure 4.16):

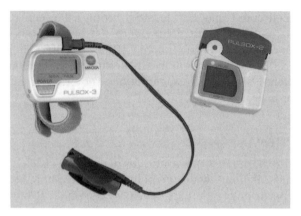

Figure 4.16. Pulse oximeters available

- Oxygen saturation
- Pulse rate
- Plethysmographic waveform

Pulse oximetry is performed with a sensor probe attached to the patient's fingertip (most common site) or earlobe. It functions by emitting red and infrared light respectively. Detectors situated on the lower side of the probe receive the light transmitted through the body tissue. The percentage of haemoglobin saturated with oxygen is calculated from the relative amounts of light that reach the detectors. While pulse oximeters are very useful and reasonably accurate, they are prone to error if used incorrectly. Any factors that reduce the perfusion of the site where the probe is positioned or that impede the passage of light through body tissue will influence the accuracy of the reading (Allen, 2004). Some factors that may reduce the accuracy of results are as follows:

- Incorrect positioning of the probe or excessive movement such as shivering or tumour will reduce the accuracy (Booker, 2004b).
- Dark-coloured nail varnish will affect the amount of light passing through the probe (Carroll, 1997).
- Bright overhead lighting or direct sunlight on the sensor can dilute the light signal from the oximeter (Allen, 2004).
- Intravenous (IV) dyes used in haemodynamic and diagnostic testing may depress readings, as they may alter light transmission. The same is possible if the patient has high bilirubin levels when jaundiced (Allen, 2004).
- Poor peripheral circulation and cold hands will give unreliable readings (Woodrow, 2000).

- Cardiac arrhythmias, especially irregular rates, will reduce the accuracy.
- Carbon monoxide poisoning causes falsely high readings (Hampson, 1998).
- High levels of carboxyhaemoglobin due to smoking causes falsely high readings (Esmond, 2001).

Although pulse oximetry offers many benefits, it is only valuable if used in conjunction with a comprehensive respiratory assessment. It is also important to remember that pulse oximeters do not provide information regarding carbon dioxide levels or pH, which are particularly relevant in the management of patients with COPD in respiratory failure. In these cases arterial blood gas analysis is required to provide a full picture of the patient's respiratory status.

Arterial Blood Gas Analysis

Arterial blood gas analysis allows the objective evaluation of a patient's oxygenation, ventilation and acid–base balance (Coombs, 2001), which can reveal vital information regarding a patient's respiratory status. Arterial blood gases are measured by taking a sample of blood from a peripheral artery, usually the radial artery. Measurements are made of the concentrations of oxygen, carbon dioxide, plasma, pH and bicarbonate levels. The normal concentration of oxygen in arterial blood (PaO_2) is 10–13 kPa, carbon dioxide ($PaCO_2$) is 4.5–6.0 kPa, pH is 7.35–7.45 and the bicarbonate level is 22–26 meq/L. An oxygen concentration of less than 8 kPa is called hypoxia. A carbon dioxide concentration of greater than 6.5 kPa is called hypercapnia.

Measurement of arterial blood gases should be considered in patients with severe disease with oxygen saturations of less than 92%, in particular if presenting with increasing symptoms of breathlessness, ankle oedema, central cyanosis and persistent low oxygen saturations. The GOLD guidelines suggest that arterial blood gases are measured in patients whose FEV_1 is less than 40% predicted or with clinical signs suggestive of respiratory failure, particularly during an exacerbation or symptoms of right heart failure. An acid–base imbalance can be an indicator for life-saving interventions and treatments such as oxygen therapy, hydration and noninvasive ventilation (NIV).

SUMMARY

Although spirometry is the gold standard for COPD and is the only accurate method of measuring the degree of airflow obstruction in patients with COPD, it should be used in conjunction with a good history and physical examination. A diagnosis of airflow obstruction can be made if $FEV_1/FVC < 70\%$ and $FEV_1 < 80\%$ predicted normal values. However, it is essential that spirometry is carried out competently by the practitioner and that the patient gives maximum effort while performing this procedure. If the patient's diagnosis remains uncertain further investigations should be completed and a specialist opinion sought to exclude other pathology.

Chapter 5

Nonpharmacological Management of Patients with COPD

INTRODUCTION

Although COPD has no cure due to the permanent damage that the lungs have incurred, there are various nonpharmacological options available in the management of COPD. The most important thing patients can do to help themselves and slow down the decline in their lung function is to stop smoking. Smoking cessation advice is therefore an essential element of nonpharmacological management in helping patients to quit. Health promotion issues such as the importance of adequate daily exercise and a balanced diet are also essential aspects of caring and managing patients with COPD.

The value of deep breathing exercises, particularly in patients prone to hyperventilation and anxiety attacks, is also significant in helping patients cope with breathlessness and are discussed in some detail. Nonpharmacological management options are just as important as pharmacological options and should be carefully thought about in the overall management of patients with COPD.

SMOKING CESSATION

Cigarette Smoking and COPD

Smoking is the single greatest cause of preventable illness and premature deaths in the UK. For patients with COPD smoking is the main cause, which affects 20% of people with a smoking history of 15–20 pack years. Smoking cessation is therefore the most effective and most important intervention to prevent further progression of COPD and decline in FEV_1. In 'at-risk' smokers the rate of decline is around 50–60 ml a year compared to healthy nonsmokers, where the rate of decline is reduced by half, to around 25–30 ml a year. Why some smokers are affected more than others, and as a result suffer an accelerated decline in their lung function, is not clearly understood. As demonstrated by Fletcher and Peto (1977), if patients manage to stop smoking, the rate of lung function decline reverts to normal over time, although the lost lung function cannot be regained. However, some patients who have smoked excessively and give up may still experience a decline in their condition and an increase in their symptoms, although the process of course will not be as rapid (Boyars, 1988).

In 1997 there were more than 11 million regular smokers in the UK, which equates to about 27% of the adult population (National Institute for Clinical Excellence, 2002). The proportions remain higher in men than women and are particularly higher within the lower socioeconomic groups. Within the younger generation 25% of 15 year olds are regular smokers (National Institute for Clinical Excellence, 2002). Smoking does not only cause COPD but also other related diseases, such as lung cancer, cardiovascular disease and peripheral vascular disease, which costs the NHS £1500 million per year to treat these patients. It is known that about 120000 smokers die prematurely each year as a result (National Institute for Clinical Excellence, 2002), which could be avoided if patients gave up. Life expectancy is also reduced compared to patients who do not smoke by about 8 years for those under the age of 35 years (National Institute for Clinical Excellence, 2002). Because of this, smoking cessation is now recognised as a top healthcare priority at both national and local levels. UK regulations have led to a reduction in the tar yield of cigarettes from 25–35 mg in the 1950s to 5–15 mg in the 1990s, with an upper limit of 12 mg set from 1997 (McLoughlin, 2005). In 1998, the Department of Health (DoH) published *Smoking Kills, A White Paper on Tobacco*, which supported the development of specialist smoking services across the UK. From 2003 to 2006 an estimated £138 m has been available to support these services by the government (Department of Health, 2003). More recently the government has also taken measures to reduce the prevalence of smoking, including action to stop tobacco advertising and promotion and banning smoking in public places and the work place. Currently, the government spends £30 m on antismoking campaigns and £41 m on smoking cessation services (ASH, 2005). The government targets aim to see 1.5 million people stop smoking by 2010 (McLoughlin, 2005).

Nicotine is the main constituent of smoke that causes addiction. Nicotine itself is not a major primary cause of smoking-related disease, but it has marked effects on arterial tone. The main disease-causing element from smoking comes from 'tar', a dark viscous fluid from tobacco smoke, which contains at least 4000 different chemicals, including over 50 known carcinogens and metabolic poisons (National Institute for Chemical Excellence, 2002). The poisonous elements in smoke, such as carbon monoxide, oxides of nitrogen and hydrogen cyanide, are largely responsible for cardiovascular disease.

Most smokers start as teenagers and continue to do so into adulthood. Due to the addiction to nicotine, most smokers find it very hard to stop. For patients who smoke it is not only an addictive habit but a conditioning response. Smoking a cigarette is often associated with everyday activities such as having a cup of tea or coffee and from a smoker's perception enables them to relax after a meal or watching television, even though in the true sense nicotine is a stimulant.

A cigarette has 0.7–1 g of tobacco, of which 1–6 mg of nicotine is inhaled directly to the lungs. A number of variables such as depth and length of inhalation, type of tobacco and methods of preparation affect the delivery of nicotine to the lungs (Croghan, 2005) and plasma levels. Following inhalation of a cigarette the transfer of nicotine across the blood–brain barrier takes as little as 7 seconds to peak. Nicotine is metabolised mainly in the liver and excreted in the urine as continine (Croghan, 2005), with some metabolism occurring in the lungs and brain (Royal College of Physicians, 2000). Nicotine has a half-life of 90–120 minutes; therefore during the course of the day, depending on the number of cigarettes smoked, the plasma concentration increases to reach 20–40 ng/ml (Royal College of Physicians, 2000).

Role of the Health Profesional in Helping Smokers Quit

Encouraging patients to stop smoking is a vital part of our role as health professionals. This is not only to reduce the costs associated with diseases caused by smoking but also to provide individual health gains. Therefore, at every available opportunity smoking cessation should be addressed and the health benefits of stopping explained to patients. Providing support in the form of one-to-one counselling or group therapy combined with nicotine replacement therapy (NRT) is the most effective and increases smoking cessation rates.

The benefit of stopping smoking begins almost immediately, with blood pressure and pulse returning to normal. Over 24 hours the carbon monoxide levels are eliminated from the body and the lungs start to clear out mucus and other smoking debris. By 3–9 months breathing problems improve, with an improvement in lung function of about 10%. After 5 years the risk of heart attack falls to half that of a smoker and after 10 years the risk of lung cancer falls to half that of a smoker. Smokers who quit before the age of 35 years can expect a life expectancy only slightly less than that of a nonsmoker. Even cessation in middle age improves health and subsequently reduces the risk of early death (National Institute for Clinical Excellence, 2002). It is important to inform all patients, no matter how many years they have smoked, that it is never too late to give up. Quitting at any age will provide both immediate and long-term health benefits.

Although about 80% of smokers express a desire to stop, only 35% attempt to do so each year, with fewer than 10% being successful (Scholey and Moss, 2005). To be successful, smokers must be motivated and want to stop smoking and believe that stopping will improve their health and life. Most smokers will have several attempts before they succeed. Therefore education in the form of leaflets and information, and support from the health professional, plays a very important role in helping patients to succeed. Government research suggests that smokers are four times more likely to quit with the help of their local NHS Stop Smoking Service, using NRT or bupropion, than if they rely on willpower alone (Department of Health, 2004b).

Intervention Steps for Health Professionals to Take

At every opportunity health professionals should approach the subject with all patients regarding their smoking history. This can be a time consuming and sometimes a frustrating task, but is an extremely valuable use of a health professional's time. The subject should be approached sensitively and in a nonthreatening manner, and preferably should not be the first question raised, to avoid giving the impression that the focus of the meeting is solely based on this subject. If health professionals approach this subject in an abrupt and threatening manner or lecture the patient about the harmful effects of smoking the patient is likely to be defensive and resist any advice that is offered. However, a supportive approach may encourage the 'contented smoker' or a smoker who is 'contemplating' giving up seriously to consider stopping (Bellamy and Booker, 2003). Some patients who may have experienced a medical critical event such as a myocardial infarction or a health scare are often more likely to accept advice and support to quit smoking.

Spirometry can provide a very useful visual assessment to demonstrate to patients the relationship between their smoking habit and deterioration in their lung function in relation to the symptoms they are experiencing. Some electronic spirometers calculate the lung age from the measured and predicted FEV_1. If the FEV_1 is reduced and demonstrates that their lung age is greater than their actual age, this may be a useful incentive in trying to encourage patients to quit. Additionally, patients with mild COPD and a smoking history who present for a screening assessment and spirometry at the clinic can be given a simple explanation using the Fletcher and Peto graph (1977) of how their lung function is likely to be accelerated by smoking. This can be a useful incentive for patients to quit before too much damage occurs to their lungs.

Even though patient records may show the patient not to be a current smoker it is important to remember to continue to check on each patient's smoking status at each visit. This is to provide praise on their efforts on quitting and to give further support if required. Some patients may fail to quit or have a relapse and start smoking again. With these patients the whole process will need to be started again, tying to determine the reasons why the patient failed to quit and to work out solutions with the patient to enable them to succeed next time (Table 5.1).

The following points may be useful to follow at each patient consultation:

- Ask all smokers about their smoking habits sensitively and in a nonthreatening way.
- Find out the reasons why they smoke.
- Assess whether patients are interested in stopping smoking or have ever stopped smoking.
- Advise on the benefits of stopping and the risks to health if they continue to smoke. Provide information on NRT or bupropion to enable patients to decide which product they would like to try.
- Provide a contact telephone number of the local NHS Stop Smoking Service or make a referral for the patient. If the patient is house-bound many local services will arrange to conduct a home visit to provide the patient with support and advice.
- If, as a health professional, you run your own smoking cessation clinics, provide the patient with an action plan and the steps to take in order to quit. Help the patient to set a quit date. Arrange for a follow-up 12 weeks later in order to provide support.

Table 5.1. Strategies to help patients quit smoking

Advise patients to dispose of all packets of tobacco or cigarettes, matches, lighters and ashtrays.
Inform their family and friends of when they plan to quit in order to provide support.
Address the hand-to-mouth ritual by distracting the hands (e.g. knitting, doodling) and mouth (e.g. chewing gum, sucking sweets, low calorie nibbles or drinking water).
Avoid mixing with people who smoke or ask if possible that they avoid smoking around the patient.
Ban smoking from their home if possible.
If a patient's partner/spouse smokes try and encourage them to quit at the same time if possible.
When out, try and sit in nonsmoking areas where possible.
Advise patients to take one day at a time.
Advise patients to alter their lifestyles and routines, particularly those with associated smoking behaviours. Keep busy and take up new activities or hobbies.
Eat a healthy diet and advise not to increase caffeine consumption as levels may rise when smoking is stopped. Avoid unhealthy or higher-calorie snacks and avoid putting excess weight on.
Take regular exercise.
Plan a series of rewards with the money saved.

• Give praise and encouragement to patients who have successfully given up. Check at each appointment that the patient has not had a relapse and started smoking again.

Withdrawal Symptoms

Withdrawal symptoms occur during periods of nonsmoking as a result of a decrease in nicotine plasma levels. As a consequence, the nicotine receptors gradually recover their active functional state and become resensitised (Scholey and Moss, 2005). As nicotine is so addictive the symptoms of withdrawal can make it difficult for some patients to continue their attempt to quit. The following symptoms should be discussed and an explanation given of why they are occurring. Therefore, the use of NRT or bupropion can help increase the chance of success. Side effects of quitting may include:

• Craving for a cigarette
• Irritability, anxiety and mood swings
• Restlessness and poor concentration
• Increased appetite

Unfortunately, for many patients who experience these symptoms the result is a failure to quit. The use of NRT products is therefore designed to assist patients to quit smoking by reducing the withdrawal symptoms and cravings for a cigarette. NRT is absorbed by the body in a different way to nicotine from cigarettes and is therefore less addictive (Percival, 2002). Although NRT does not provide an alternative for cigarettes or a replacement for will-power it enables patients to cope better with their cravings, thereby ensuring a higher success rate. Research has shown that using NRT products doubles the individual's chances of successfully succeeding in quitting (Gregory and Bason, 2003).

NRT products are available over the counter and are included in the Nurse Prescribers Formulary, and many nurses can supply NRT under patient group directives. All current NRT products (Table 5.2) have a similar success rate and patients should decide which product they feel would suit them and their lifestyle best. The main medical contraindications to NRT include cardiovascular disease, hyperthyroidism, diabetes mellitus, severe renal or hepatic impairment and peptic ulcer (National Institute for Clinical Excellence, 2002). However, within these groups of patients smoking, when providing advice, heath professionals need to weigh up the significant harm by continuing to smoke and the use of NRT.

The dosage of NRT will depend on the number of cigarettes smoked per day and the time the patient has the first cigarette of the day. NICE guidelines (National Institute for Clinical Excellence, 2002) indicate that in trials, a

Table 5.2. Nicotine replacement therapy products available. Taken from National Institute for Clinical Excellence (2002)

Nicotine transdermal patches
  5 mg, 10 mg, 15 mg (Nicorette®, Pharmacia)
  7 mg, 14 mg, 21 mg per 24 hours (Nicotinelle® TTS 10, TTS 20, TTS 30, Novartis
    Consumer Health)
  7 mg, 14 mg, 21 mg (NiQuitin CQ®, GlaxoSmith Kline)

Nicotine chewing gum
  2 mg, 4 mg (Nicorette®, Pharmacia, Nicotinell®, Novartis Consumer Health)

Nicotine 2 mg sublingual tablet (Nicotinell® Microtab, Pharmacia)

Nicotine 1 mg lozenge (Nicorette®, Novartis Consumer Health)
Nicotine 2 mg, 4 mg lozenge (NiQuitin CQ®, GlaxoSmith Kline)

Nicotine 10 mg inhalator cartridge plus mouthpiece (Nicorette® inhalator,
  Pharmacia)

Nicotine 0.5 mg per puff of metred nasal spray (Nicorette®, Pharmacia)

---

combination of two different NRT products is more likely to be effective than a single NRT product such as nicotine patches plus either gum, lozenges or inhalator to help reduce cravings. Usually a prescription is issued every 2 weeks to monitor and assess effectiveness and reduce the doses of nicotine over an 8–12 week period.

Some listed side effects of NRT include the following:

- Nausea
- Dizziness
- Headaches and cold-like symptoms
- Palpitations
- Dyspepsia
- Insomnia
- Vivid dreams
- Local reaction dependent on product used

Nicotine Replacement Products

Nicotine Patches

Nicotine patches are easy to use, and work by giving a slow release of nicotine. There are two types of patch (16 or 24 hour) and are available in several strengths. This enables the patient to reduce the strength of the patch over a 12 week programme. Occasionally the adhesive in the patches can cause local skin irritation; therefore the site should be rotated.

NICOTINE GUM

This is available in two strengths (2 and 4 mg) and a variety of flavours. The gum is chewed slowly to release the nicotine until the flavour of the gum is released, and then positioned between the check and gum to allow the nicotine to be absorbed. This sequence is repeated when the desire to smoke is felt again, a technique known as 'chew–rest–chew'. Each piece of gum lasts about 20 minutes and up to 16 pieces can be chewed in 24 hours.

NASAL SPRAY

Nicotine nasal spray is absorbed very rapidly via the nasal mucosa, reaching a peak within 10 seconds. Each spray contains 0.5 mg of nicotine and can be administered up to 64 sprays per day. It is particularly effective for highly dependent smokers or patients experiencing severe withdrawal symptoms. The spray can initially cause a sore throat or runny nose, but this soon passes within a couple of days.

SUBLINGUAL TABLET

These are placed under the tongue and dissolve slowly over a period of 20–30 minutes, releasing a controlled level of nicotine that is absorbed through the lining of the mouth. It should be emphasised to patients that these should not be sucked, chewed or swallowed, as this will reduce the effectiveness and amount of nicotine absorbed. Each tablet contains 2 mg of nicotine and up to 16 per day can be used on a regular basis.

LOZENGE

These are available in three strengths (1, 2 and 4 mg) and are used in a similar way to the gum in that the lozenge should be sucked until the taste is strong and then placed between the cheek and gum. This is repeated every few minutes for 20–30 minutes until the lozenge has dissolved completely. The nicotine is slowly absorbed through the lining of the mouth and can be repeated up to 12–15 times per day.

INHALATOR

This is a plastic device similar to a cigarette into which a nicotine cartridge fits. Each cartridge contains 10 mg of nicotine (3×20 minute sessions), which is absorbed through the lining of the mouth. The advantage of this particular device addresses the behavioural habit for smokers who miss the hand-to-mouth action. Between 6 and 12 cartridges can be used per day on a regular basis.

BUPROPION HYDROCHLORIDE

The tablet bupropion hydrochloride (Zyban) was initially developed as an antidepressant. It works by reducing the desire to smoke and reducing withdrawal symptoms. Although it has been found to be effective, like NRT, it is not a replacement for motivation and willpower to stop. The patient while still smoking sets a quit date, 2 weeks after starting the course of tablets. Dosage is 150 mg (one tablet) daily for the first six days and then increasing on day seven to 150 mg twice daily, at least 8 hours apart for 8 weeks. If the smoker fails to stop smoking after one month of treatment, he or she is unlikely to succeed and should be reviewed and treatment stopped. Bupropion is generally well tolerated, but is not suitable for everyone. Therefore a full clinical assessment should be conducted before being prescribed. Contraindications to its use include:

- Current seizure disorder or any history of seizures
- Current or previous diagnosis of bulimia or anorexia nervosa
- Known central nervous system tumour
- Undergoing withdrawal from alcohol or benzodiazepines
- Severe hepatic cirrhosis
- History of bipolar disorder (e.g. manic-depressive psychosis)

In addition, bupropion can interact with other medication, such as other antidepressants (MAOIs), antipsychotics and theophyllines, as well as over-the-counter drugs such as Nytol and St John's wort. The most common side effects include difficulty in sleeping, headaches, dizziness, dry mouth, rashes and itching.

Smoking cessation is the single most effective way of reducing the risk of developing COPD as well as to halt its progression. Spending time offering practical information, literature and support to patients who have the motivation to quit is time well spent. Remember to enquire regarding smoking status at each patient's appointment in a sensitive and nonthreatening way, even if previously they had stopped smoking, to ensure they have not started again. If patients fail, find out the reason why and encourage them to try again. Sometimes quitting with someone else provides additional incentive and support. Provide telephone help line numbers for patients to ring for support if they find cravings become hard to overcome.

OTHER NONPHARMACOLOGICAL MANAGEMENT

The Importance of Exercise

Exercise is important to maintain fitness and wellbeing. Exercise even if minimal can help keep the lungs healthy by improving lung capacity and

Chronic Obstructive Pulmonary Disease

exercise tolerance. Unfortunately, patients with COPD gradually stop exercising due to the degree of breathlessness they experience. As a result of breathlessness this eventually leads to deconditioning and patients enter the dangerous spiral of inactivity (Figure 5.1).

The less exercise patients take, the more the sensation of breathlessness on minimal exertion will be increased. Reduced activity may lead to social isolation and increased disability. This vicious circle is characteristic of patients in the advanced stages of COPD. It is therefore essential that health professionals advise patients that becoming breathless, although distressing, is not harmful to them and that regular exercise is vital to lead as normal a life as possible. Patients with COPD should be encouraged to pace themselves and

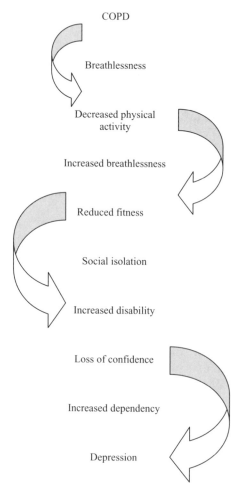

COPD

Breathlessness

Decreased physical
activity

Increased breathlessness

Reduced fitness

Social isolation

Increased disability

Loss of confidence

Increased dependency

Depression

Figure 5.1. Spiral of inactivity in patients with COPD

take regular daily exercise within the limitations of their breathlessness. This should be in the form of a daily walk when weather permits and gentle arm and leg exercises to maintain muscle tone and fitness (Table 5.3). Such an exercise programme can be built up slowly over several weeks to help increase the patient's physical exercise tolerance and stamina. Swimming is a good form of exercise, particularly for patients with breathlessness. For those who are able, joining a leisure centre can also be beneficial. Positive enforcement of the benefits of regular exercise to patients at each follow-up appointment is useful.

Management of Breathlessness

Breathlessness is the most distressing and frightening symptom of all in patients with COPD. As a result, breathlessness is commonly associated with anxiety and panic attacks, which only makes breathlessness worse and creates tension in the shoulder and neck muscles. In this situation the patient tends to take rapid shallow breaths, which are ineffective, and wastes energy instead

Table 5.3. Suggested exercise programme for patients with COPD

1. Shoulder shrugging – circle shoulders forward, down, backward and up. Repeat three times, with a short rest in between.
2. Full arm rotations – one arm at a time, pass arm as near as possible to side of head, in as large a circle as possible. Repeat three times, with a short rest in between.
3. Gentle movement of head from side to side – move head left, right, forward and back gently and slowly, repeating three times.
4. Increasing arm circles – hold one arm away from body at shoulder height and move it in a small circle for a count of six circles. Repeat with the other arm.
5. Sitting to standing – using a dining chair, sit, stand and sit, trying not to push up from the chair. Repeat continuously for 30 seconds up to a total of four repetitions.
6. Leg extensions – sitting on a dining chair, slowly straighten left knee, trying to keep back of thigh on chair, then slowly lower; repeat with right leg. Repeat exercise three times.
7. Calf exercises – stand upright, holding on to the back of a chair. Rise up on to the toes and then back to the floor. Repeat this continuously for 30 seconds.
8. Trunk side flexion – sit on a chair and reach down to the left side as far as possible, then slowly return to the centre. Repeat bending to the right. Repeat this continuously for 30 seconds.
9. Walking on the spot – stand upright, holding on to the back of a chair. Allow one knee to bend, keeping toes on the ground, and then bend other knee while straightening the first knee. Repeat this continuously for 30 seconds.
10. Step-ups – stand at the bottom of the stairs. With one foot step up and then down, repeating the process with the other foot. Repeat this continuously for 30 seconds.

Advise patients to repeat this set of exercises at least three times a week.

of using the diaphragm. As a result, the lungs are not emptied as well as normal, so there is a greater amount of air in the lungs at the end of expiration. Hyperinflation of the lungs with air-trapping in the alveoli leads to increased residual volume, and less space is available for the inspiratory volume of the next breath. Patients feel as if they are blowing up like a balloon, gasping but unable to force any more air into their overinflated lungs.

The aims of breathlessness management are therefore to reduce the work of breathing and to give patients confidence in their ability to control their breathless attacks. Correct breathing techniques can increase breathing efficiency, which helps minimise the trapped air and the uncomfortable feelings of breathlessness. The following steps may be initiated to help re-educate the patient and manage their breathlessness:

1. The most important thing is to get the patient to adopt a comfortable position, by sitting upright in a chair (Figure 5.2), leaning forward (Figure 5.3), standing upright against a wall (Figure 5.4) or leaning over the back of a chair or a stable object (Figure 5.5). These positions help support the shoulders and the upper chest to relax and allow the diaphragm and abdomen to expand.
2. Encourage patients to pay particular attention to their breathing patterns. Do they breathe through their nose or mouth? Do they use just the upper part of their chest or abdomen? Are they pursed-lip breathing?
3. Next, encourage patients to be aware of any tension present in their neck, jaw or shoulder muscles. If tension is present gentle shoulder shrugging or massage of the muscles will help. Re-educating patients to reduce the work of breathing will in time reduce the amount of muscle tension.

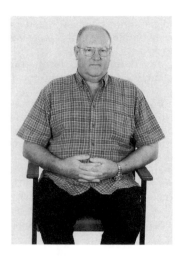

Figure 5.2. Sitting upright in a chair

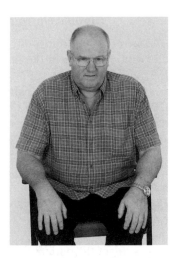

Figure 5.3. Leaning forward in a chair

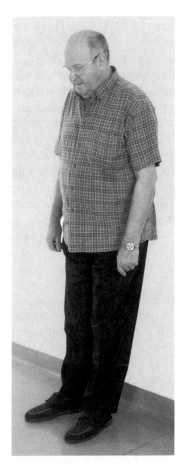

Figure 5.4. Standing against a wall

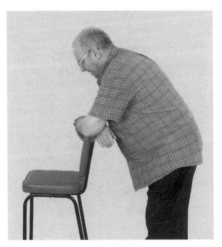

Figure 5.5. Leaning over the back of a chair

4. When the patient is comfortable and relaxed encourage him or her to adopt the abdominal breathing technique. This will take time and practice, but should be encouraged until the patient is familiar with the breathing pattern. Once taught patients can be encouraged to incorporate it into their daily activities and daily exercise. Pursed-lip breathing is often adopted voluntary by patients with breathlessness as it helps maintain air pressure in the small airways, preventing them from collapsing. However, with breathing re-education patients may find it unnecessary, although this should not be discouraged if pursed-lip breathing helps patients relieve their breathlessness. Once a comfortable position has been adopted and patients are relaxed, they should practice abdominal breathing by placing their hands on their abdomen and follow the instructions below:

- Encourage patients to breathe out gently like a sigh. Inhale a deep breath, allowing the abdomen to rise and as they exhale allowing their abdomen to fall. After each breath pause for 1–2 seconds before breathing again. Repeat this exercise five times per session, several times a day. It may help if patients close their eyes or listen to some relaxing music to help them relax and concentrate.
- Whenever patients experience a breathless attack, explain that they should keep calm and take up one of the positions they find comfortable. They should be encouraged to try and relax and breathe using the abdominal breathing technique, trying to take slow gentle breaths until they regain control. Encourage patients to focus mentally on a pleasant image or to adapt a phase that they can repeat in their minds. It is important for patients to find out what works for them.

Hopefully, by patients learning to control their breathlessness rather than the breathlessness controlling them they will reduce their anxiety and panic attacks and will learn to cope and fell less frightened. It may also be useful to have a member of the family present when teaching the patient abdominal breathing in order to enforce and help the patient when these breathless attacks occur. Patients will therefore feel much more confident and will ensure they keep active and enjoy a better quality of life.

NUTRITION IN COPD

Adequate nutrition is an important aspect of management for patients with COPD. Many patients with advanced COPD, usually with emphysema, are underweight and even cachectic. Other patients, usually with chronic bronchitis, are more likely to be overweight. During a patient's assessment details of the dietary intake and measurement of the body mass index (BMI) should be included. The objective is not simply to identify patients at risk, but those who despite an adequate dietary intake are also losing weight (Table 5.4).

Weight loss in many patients with COPD is due to a number of factors. This is usually as a consequence of reduced dietary intake due to their breathlessness or altered absorption if hypoxic. As a result of the work of increased breathing, resting energy expenditure is also increased (Schols and Wouters, 2000). However, a sudden and significant weight loss should raise suspicions of other underlying causes such as malignancy, tuberculosis or hyperthyroidism. Recent studies on malnutrition in COPD have looked at the

Table 5.4. Calculation of the body mass index (BMI) and a BMI assessment chart

$$BMI = \frac{weight\ (in\ kg)}{(height)^2\ (in\ metres)}$$

Example:

$$BMI = \frac{61}{1.75 \times 1.75} = 19.9$$

BMI assessment chart	
BMI	Nutritional status
<16	Severe malnourishment
16–18.5	Moderate malnourishment
18.5–21	At risk
21–25	Ideal
25–30	Moderate obesity
>30	Severe obesity

consequences of weight loss, particularly whether it is an independent predictor of outcome and whether interventions are effective both at increasing weight and influencing outcome (National Collaborating Centre for Chronic Conditions, 2004). A low BMI is suggestive of a poor prognosis (Landbo *et al.*, 1999), especially in those with advanced disease, while an increase in BMI with treatment improves prognosis (Schols *et al.*, 1998). Malnutrition affects the composition and function of respiratory muscle and impairs skeletal muscle function, affecting exercise performance of these patients.

Dietary Requirements for Patients with COPD

A healthy and varied diet, following the Mediterranean diet, in particular wholegrains, fresh fruit and vegetables, is beneficial in slowing down the progression of COPD (Collins, 2003). Although public health campaigns encourage people to eat at least five portions of fruit and vegetables daily, the average consumption in the UK is three portions, increasing the risk of COPD (Watson *et al.*, 2002). It is unclear whether this benefit is derived from the fruit's vitamin and mineral content, the presence of antioxidant phytochemicals or anti-inflammatory substances (Collins, 2003). However, it is thought that high levels of antioxidants in vitamins C and E have a protective effect on lung tissue. Some natural fish oils may also protect the lungs through antioxidant enhancement (Bellamy and Booker, 2003), but there is insufficient evidence to support this claim.

Protein requirements are variable depending on the COPD severity and presence of infection. A patient with a low BMI, which is common in end-stage COPD, is often associated with abnormal protein metabolism. Patients in this group therefore require double the normal protein intake of 1.5 g/kg daily (Sauerwein and Romijn, 1999).

Osteoporosis is common in patients with advanced COPD (Biskobing, 2002), as a result of poor dietary intake, reduced absorption and altered bone remodelling rates due to limited weight-bearing activity, compounded by steroid use (Gagnon *et al.*, 1997). The National Osteoporosis Society states that calcium supplements should be offered to all COPD patients with proven osteoporosis, to increase total calcium intake to 1200 mg a day (Collins, 2003).

For patients with a low BMI, nutritional supplements to increase their total calorific intake may prove beneficial and have been shown to improve survival (National Collaborating Centre for Chronic Conditions, 2004). However, there are no additional benefits in patients who are not underweight (Halpin, 2003).

Dietary Advice for Patients

- Eat a healthy balanced diet.
- Eat little and often, particularly if eating increases the sensation of breathlessness.

- Patients who are overweight should be advised to lose weight and increase their daily exercise.
- Avoid gas-forming vegetables such as beans, cabbage and peppers, which can lead to abdominal distension and diaphragmatic splinting, causing increased breathlessness (Halpin, 2003).
- Reduce the amount of dairy produce in the diet if prone to producing large amounts of sputum.

Chapter 6

Pharmacological Management of Patients with Stable COPD

INTRODUCTION

As previously discussed in Chapter 4, an early and accurate diagnosis is essential, particularly in those patients over the age of 35 and at high risk with a smoking history of 20 pack years. Ultimately the overall aims of management of stable COPD is to ensure good control of symptoms, to slow down the progression of the disease and to prevent further deterioration or complications. The sooner the diagnosis is made and interventions implemented, the more the long-term prognosis is improved. Interventions to control symptoms include pharmacology treatments such as inhaled or nebulised bronchodilator therapy, corticosteroid therapy, short-burst oxygen therapy and miscellaneous therapy including influenza and pneumococcus vaccinations. These treatments and the various inhalers available will be discussed in turn.

INHALED BRONCHODILATOR THERAPY

Although COPD is characterised by irreversible airflow obstruction, bronchodilators are the mainstay of drug therapy in COPD (British Thoracic Society, 1997b). There are three classes of bronchodilator therapies available to treat patients with COPD, including beta-2 agonists, anticholinergics and oral theophyllines.

Beta-2 agonists act directly on bronchial smooth muscle to cause bronchodilation whereas anticholinergics act by inhibiting resting broncho-motor tone (National Collaborating Centre for Chronic Conditions, 2004). As a result both drugs affect the degree of breathlessness, which is improved by increasing exercise tolerance. Although they do not significantly improve FEV_1, bronchodilators can reduce air-trapping, improve the efficiency of respiratory muscles and reduce symptoms of breathlessness on exertion (Booker, 2005).

Both anticholinergic and beta-2 agonist bronchodilators are useful in COPD. Anticholinergics appear more useful in the relief of symptoms in older patients or those with severe disease and a heavy smoking history (Braun *et al.*, 1989). In order to rationalise management and treatment, the responsiveness of individual patients should be assessed both objectively with measurements of lung function and also by asking the patient if they have noticed any improvements in symptoms, activities of living, exercise capacity and rapidity of symptom relief (Table 6.1). If the patient remains symptomatic or experiences two or more exacerbations per year then long-acting bronchodilators should be considered. Any new treatment that is introduced should be for a trial period and the benefits and effectiveness evaluated. If no improvement or benefit is seen then the inhaler should be stopped and further options considered.

Short-Acting Beta-2 Agonists

Short-acting beta-2 agonists are the most commonly used bronchodilators in COPD. Short-acting beta-2 agonists such as salbutamol (Ventolin®, Salamol®, Asmasal®) and terbutaline (Bricanyl®) have a rapid onset of action and are useful for obtaining prompt relief of symptoms. They act directly on bronchial smooth muscle to cause bronchodilation, lasting up to four hours. For maximum effect and to sustain bronchodilation they are recommended to be taken four times daily and 'as required' for relief of breathlessness. It may also be beneficial to advise the patient to use a short-acting beta-2 agonist prior to exercise in order to increase exercise tolerance and reduce the degree of breathlessness during the activity. Short-acting beta-2 agonists are widely used as first-line therapy for patients with COPD and are usually used in combination with anticholinergic bronchodilators.

Long-Acting Beta-2 Agonists

Long-acting beta-2 agonists have a similar action to short-acting bronchodilators but they have a longer onset of action and duration of 12 hours. The two long-acting beta-2 agonists, salmeterol (Serevent®) and formoterol (Foradil®, Oxis®), are both licensed for use in COPD and are administered twice daily.

Table 6.1. Assessing the effectiveness of drug treatment. Taken from Jones (2001)

Has their treatment made a difference to them?
Has their breathing become easier in any way?
Can they do some things now that they could not do before, or the same things but faster?
Are they able to do the same things as before but are less breathless doing them?
Has their sleep improved?

In the treatment of COPD, long-acting beta-2 agonists have been shown to improve health status and breathlessness scores (Jones and Bosh, 1997). Salmeterol has also been shown to improve breathlessness at night (Bellamy and Booker, 2003). Long-acting beta-2 agonists also appear to reduce the frequency of exacerbations of moderate to severe COPD, particularly when given in combination with high doses of inhaled corticosteroids (Calverly *et al.*, 2003). Mahler *et al.* (1999) also demonstrated in a study an increase between exacerbations when compared with a placebo and ipratropium bromide.

CONTRAINDICATIONS (for full details see the most recent edition of the British National Formulary (BNF) or the Summary of Product Characteristics (SPC) for the relevant preparation)

Beta-2 agonists should be used with caution in patients with the following conditions (British National Formulary, 2005):

- Hypersensitivity
- Tachydysrhythmias
- Severe heart disease
- Heart block

CAUTIONS (for full details see the most recent edition of the BNF or the SPC for the relevant preparation)

Beta-2 agonists should be used with caution in patients with the following conditions (British National Formulary, 2005):

- Hyperthyroidism
- Cardiovascular disease
- Arrhythmias
- Hypertension
- Diabetes

In high doses there is an increased risk of hypokalaemia, particularly if used at more than the standard dose. This may also be potentiated if given with high-dose corticosteroids, potassium-sparing diuretics or theophylline.

ADVERSE EFFECTS (for full details see the most recent edition of the BNF or the SPC for the relevant preparation)

Generally beta-2 agonists are well tolerated and cause few problems when used in standard doses. Side effects that may occur are (British National Formulary, 2005):

- Tremor
- Palpitations
- Anxiety
- Tachycardia
- Nausea
- Irritation of the throat

Short-Acting Anticholinergics

Anticholinergic drugs cause smooth muscle relaxation and bronchodilation by blocking the bronchoconstrictor effect exerted by cholinergic nerves within the lungs (Halpin, 2004). Increased bronchomotor tone is thought to be an important component of airflow obstruction in COPD (Booker, 2004a). Anticholinergic drugs are therefore beneficial in patients with COPD. Ipratropium bromide (Atrovent®), the anticholinergic agent used in the treatment of COPD, has a slower onset of action of 30–45 minutes and is therefore not suitable for rapid symptom relief or 'as-required' administration. Its effects last six hours and it is generally used regularly four times daily.

Long-Acting Anticholinergics

Tiotropium bromide (Spiriva®) is a new anticholinergic agent and has a 24 hour duration of action. In clinical trials involving patients with COPD, tiotropium bromide demonstrated a significant increase in FEV_1 and FVC compared to ipratropium bromide (Casaburi *et al.*, 2002) and reduced frequency of exacerbations (Brusasco *et al.*, 2003). A further study demonstrated greater improvements in health status and quality of life using St George's Respiratory Questionnaire when compared to ipratropium (Vincken *et al.*, 2002).

Tiotropium bromide is formulated as a capsule containing 18 µg of tiotropium as a dry powder, which is delivered using an inhaler known as the Handihaler®.

CAUTIONS (for full details see the most recent edition of the BNF or the SPC for the relevant preparation)

Anticholinergics should be used with caution in patients with the following conditions (British National Formulary, 2005):

- Prostatic hypertrophy
- Glaucoma (patient's eyes should be protected from nebulised drug or from dry powder)
- Bladder outflow obstruction

ADVERSE EFFECTS   (for full details see the most recent edition of the BNF or the SPC for the relevant preparation)

Inhaled anticholinergic agents are usually well tolerated. The most common side effects are (British National Formulary, 2005):

- Dry mouth
- Urinary retention
- Constipation
- Headache
- Nausea

Combined Short-Acting Inhaled Therapy

A combination of a short-acting beta-2 agonist and anticholinergic (Combivent®) is used four times daily. These two classes of drug work well in combination and may produce better bronchodilation than either agent used on its own in patients with COPD. Combined therapy may produce greater improvements in exercise tolerance and a greater degree of bronchodilation than either drug used separately (Bellamy and Booker, 2003).

Combined therapy can be extremely useful in patients who have sight problems and may get mixed up with too many different inhalers. Also in patients who have a tendency to forget to use their inhaler the use of a combined inhaler may be more convenient and increase compliance. The drawback of combination inhalers is the loss of flexibility in dosing of component drugs in the inhaler (Booker, 2004a).

THEOPHYLLINE

Theophylline and its derivatives have been used for many years to treat patients with COPD. They are used as a third-line treatment in patients with COPD (National Collaborating Centre for Chronic Conditions, 2004) to relieve the symptoms of breathlessness. Theophylline should therefore only be used when other inhaled bronchodilators, both short- and long-acting, have been optimised or in patients who are not able to use inhaled therapy. However, theophyllines are relatively ineffective bronchodilators and only a small number of patients obtain full benefit. Most patients appear to experience adverse side effects.

The mechanism of action of these drugs remains uncertain (Vassallo and Lipsky, 1998) but their mode of action is thought to induce relaxation of the smooth muscle in the airways. Theophylline also appears to increase diaphragmatic strength in patients with COPD (Murciano *et al.*, 1984), and this may improve ventilation and delay the onset of fatigue. Theophylline has effects on mucociliary clearance (Ziment, 1987) as well as extra pulmonary effects, particularly improvements in cardiac output (Matthay and Mahler, 1986).

CAUTIONS   (for full details see the most recent edition of the BNF or the SPC for the relevant preparation)

Theophylline should be used with caution in the elderly and in patients with the following conditions (British National Formulary, 2005):

- Cardiac disease
- Hypertension
- Hyperthyroidism
- Peptic ulcer
- Hepatic impairment
- Epilepsy
- Monitor potassium

The risks and benefits need to be considered carefully and the benefits measured both in terms of improvements in lung function or improvements in symptoms, exercise tolerance and quality of life. A trial period is suggested and the benefits, if any, evaluated. Due to possible differences in bioavailability of preparations available, theophyllines should be prescribed by their proprietary name.

ADVERSE EFFECTS   (for full details see the most recent edition of the BNF or the SPC for the relevant preparation)

The main problems with theophylline use are toxicity and potential interactions with other drugs. Therefore they require careful prescribing and monitoring of plasma concentrations. A serum level of 10–20 mg per litre (known as the therapeutic window) is necessary to be effective and produce satisfactory bronchodilation. The most common side effects are (British National Formulary, 2005):

Gastrointestinal

- Nausea
- Vomiting
- Other gastrointestinal disturbances

Neurological

- Headache
- Insomnia
- Convulsions

Cardiovascular

- Palpitations
- Tachycardia
- Cardiac arrhythmias

Interactions

As theophylline is metabolised in the liver absorption is particularly affected in patients with hepatic impairment, heart failure or if taken with certain drugs (Table 6.2). The half-life is increased in heart failure, cirrhosis, viral infections and elderly patients and by drugs such as cimetidine, ciprofloxacin, erthromycin and fluvoxamine (British National Formulary, 2005). The half-life of theophyllines is decreased in smokers and in chronic alcoholism and by drugs such as pheytoin, carbamazepine, rifampicin and barbiturates (British National Formulary, 2005).

INHALED CORTICOSTEROID THERAPY

The appropriate role of inhaled corticosteroids in COPD is controversial. It is understood that COPD, like asthma, is associated with inflammation. However, the pattern of inflammation and the response to corticosteroids are different. In COPD there is a greater number of macrophages and cytotoxic T-lymphocytes in the small airways and lung parenchyma, and an increase in macrophages and neutrophils within the sputum. The inflammation in asthma is characterised by thickening of the basement membrane as well as an increase in eosinophils and activation of mast and T-helper lymphocytes,

Table 6.2. Factors affecting serum theophylline levels. Taken from British National Formulary (2005)

Increase theophylline levels	Decrease theophylline levels
Drugs	Drugs
Cimetidine and famotidine	Furosemide
Erythromycin and ciprofloxacin	Phenytoin and carbamazepine
Fluvoxamine	Rifampicin
Diltiazem and verapamil	Barbiturates
Other factors	Other factors
Smoking cessation	Smoking
Cor pulmonale	Excessive alcohol consumption
Hepatic impairment	
Heart failure	
Viral infections	
Influenza vaccination	

which are characteristic of asthma (Jeffery, 1998). Nevertheless, there is little evidence to suggest that inhaled steroids have any effect on the inflammatory cells present in COPD as neutrophils, unlike eosinophils, are relatively insensitive to the effects of steroids (Halpin, 2003). Even high doses of inhaled steroids do not decrease the number of inflammatory cells or the level of cytokines (Keatings *et al.*, 1997). However, there appears to be some evidence showing a reduction in exacerbation rates in patients treated with inhaled steroids.

Long-Term Clinical Trials of Inhaled Corticosteroids in COPD

Various clinical trials have examined the use of long-term inhaled steroids with a placebo on the progression of COPD. These studies did not produce a sustained reduction in the rate of lung function decline at any stage of COPD and did not have any benefit in cases of mild disease (Pauwels *et al.*, 1999; Vestbo *et al.*, 1999), although in patients with moderate to severe COPD inhaled steroids did appear to reduce the number of exacerbations and improve the quality of life (Burge *et al.*, 2000).

- The EuroSCOP Study (Pauwels *et al.*, 1999) was a large European study, which investigated patients with mild COPD and compared budesonide 800 μg daily with a placebo over a 3 year period. There was no significant change in the rate of decline in FEV_1. Initially, in the first 3 months the results demonstrated some improvement with the budesonide, followed by a similar decline in FEV_1 to that within the placebo group, revealing limited long-term benefit on the rate of decline in lung function.
- The Copenhagen Lung Study (Vestbo *et al.*, 1999) was a 3 year Danish study comparing budesonide 800 μg daily with a placebo. This group of patients had mild asthma. At the end of the study, the decline in FEV_1 was almost identical, indicating no significant benefit from budesonide.
- The ISOLDE Study (Burge *et al.*, 2000) was a British study, which investigated a more severe group of patients with more severe COPD over a 3 year period using fluticasone 500 μg twice daily. The results revealed no effect on the rate of decline in lung function between the two groups. However, there were some improvements in the patient's quality of life. Patients receiving fluticasone had a significantly slower rate of decline in health status than the placebo group and the exacerbation rate was lower.
- The Lung Health 11 Study (Lung Health Study Research Group, 2000) was a large study from the USA, which investigated patients with mild to moderate COPD, treated with triamcinolone 600 μg (this formulation is not available in the UK) or a placebo over a 3 year period. As with the other studies, there was no effect on the rate of decline of FEV_1 between the two groups. However, patients in the triamcinolone group reported fewer respiratory symptoms and fewer medical consultations.

- Inhaled corticosteroid meta-analysis (Van Grunsven *et al.*, 1999) was a combined Dutch–French study, which looked at the effects of inhaled steroids over a control group using a placebo over a 2 year period. The patients using inhaled steroids were divided into two groups, one using beclometasone 1500μg daily and another group using a lower dose of budesonide, 800μg daily. The group using the high-dose steroids demonstrated a small improvement of FEV_1 during the two years of treatment, although there was no difference in exacerbation rates in the two groups.

NICE Guidelines Advice on Inhaled Corticosteroids in COPD

NICE guidelines (National Collaborating Centre for Chronic Conditions, 2004) recommend that inhaled steroids used in the management of COPD should be reserved for patients whose FEV_1 is less than 50% of the predicted value and who have experienced two or more exacerbations in the previous 12 months. The aim of the treatment is to reduce exacerbation rates and slow the decline in health status rather than to improve lung function. This recommendation is based largely on the ISOLDE trial in which subjects with a mean FEV_1 of 50% of predicted normal value had a 25% reduction in frequency of exacerbations when treated with inhaled fluticasone propionate. Exacerbations appear to accelerate the rate of lung function decline in COPD (Donaldson *et al.*, 2002). In addition, the reduction in exacerbations demonstrated in the ISOLDE trial supports the use of inhaled steroids to reduce the frequency in exacerbations independently of the drug's effects on underlying airway inflammation (Sutherland and Cherniack, 2004).

The guidelines, however, do not provide any guidance with regard to the recommended inhaled steroid or the suggested optimum dose. Currently none of the inhaled corticosteroid available is licensed for use alone in the treatment of COPD, although combination inhalers such as Symbicort® 400/12 Turbohaler® (budesonide 400μg and formoterol fumarate 12μg) and Seretide 500 Accuhaler® (fluticasone propionate 500μg and salmeterol 50μg) are licensed for COPD. The study by Burge *et al.* (2000), on which the NICE guideline recommendations are also based, uses 1000μg of fluticasone propionate daily. Studies by Calverley *et al.* (2003) and Szafranski *et al.* (2003) showed similar beneficial effects using Symbicort® (budesonide 800μg daily) and Seretide® (fluticasone propionate 1000μg) despite differing doses of inhaled steroid. GOLD (Global Initiative for Chronic Obstructive Lung Disease, 2003) notes that corticosteroids combined with long-acting beta-2 agonists are more effective than components alone.

Adverse Effects

It is important to consider the risk of side effects of inhaled steroids balanced against the benefits, especially in elderly patients. As it is difficult to predict which patients may benefit from inhaled steroid therapy both clinical and spirometry responses should be assessed to establish whether any benefit has been gained. If no substantial clinical or physiological improvement is seen, the treatment should be discontinued, since there is no evidence that continuing such treatment has any long-term benefits (Sutherland and Cherniack, 2004).

Patients with COPD are at particular risk of systemic effects of inhaled steroids, in particular osteoporosis, cataracts, skin bruising or thinning and glaucoma. Local adverse effects may also include oral candidiasis, dysphonia (which may be minimised by reminding patients to rinse their mouths with water after use), cough and bronchoconstriction. The Lung Health 11 Study also showed a reduction in bone density in the lumber spine and femur in the patients treated with triamcinolone. Hubbard *et al.* (2002) reported, in a population-based case-control study, an association with a dose-related increase in hip fractures in patients using inhaled steroids.

ORAL STEROIDS

The NICE guidelines (National Collaborating Centre for Chronic Conditions, 2004) do not recommend the use of a trial of oral steroid reversibility testing, except when it may be useful in detecting a coexisting chronic asthmatic component to their disease. It is a poor predictor of the response to inhaled steroids in patients with COPD and should therefore not be used to identify which patients should be prescribed inhaled steroids.

A majority of patients with COPD may require short-term courses of steroids during an exacerbation. However, small proportions of patients, especially those with severe COPD, appear to deteriorate when low doses of oral steroids are withdrawn, with worsening breathlessness, cough and wheeze. Although maintenance use of oral steroids is not recommended for long-term use in patients with COPD, such cases as described above may require a low dose to manage their symptoms. However, there is no published evidence or studies to support the long-term use of oral steroid therapy. The long-term side effects should be carefully explained to the patient who should be monitored for the development of osteoporosis and given appropriate prophylactic hormonal or bisphosphonate therapy. Patients over the age of 65 should be prescribed a bisphosphonate to reduce the risk of osteoporosis (National Collaborating Centre for Chronic Conditions, 2004).

ADVERSE EFFECTS

Oral steroids carry with them a dose and duration dependent risk of systemic side effects (McEvoy and Niewoehner, 1997). When used in the short term, patients may notice an increased appetite, dyspepsia, mood swings, insomnia and ankle oedema. With longer term or frequent high-dose treatment patients may develop skin thinning, bruise easily, weight gain, cataracts, osteoporosis, diabetes, increased susceptibility to infection and hypertension (British National Formulary, 2005).

INHALER DEVICES

Hand-held inhaler devices are an effective and efficient method of administering medication when used correctly by patents with COPD. They are certainly cheaper and more convenient for patients to use on a daily basis than a nebuliser. However, it is important that the correct inhaler device is provided to the patient and that they understand how to use them correctly. Inhalers require a degree of manual dexterity and some require good 'hand–breath' coordination. Therefore, when considering delivery devices, coexisting problems such as arthritis and cognitive impairment may need to be taken into account (Table 6.3).

To ensure the drug is inhaled effectively, a good inhaler technique is essential in order to reach the peripheral airways rather than the drug being deposited in the mouth and pharynx. For adequate drug deposition within the peripheral airways, particle sizes of 2–5 μm need to be produced. To achieve maximum particle deposition involves several mechanisms, which dictate how an inhaler device should be used. Breathing the aerosol in slowly and deeply reduces the amount of impact in the mouth and pharynx and allows the particles to travel into the smaller airways. Holding one's breath after slowly inhaling the aerosol gives the particles a chance to deposit by sedimentation and diffusion. If the breath is not held, the very small particles that rely on deposition by diffusion, along with a proportion of the slightly larger particles that have not had time to settle, will be exhaled (Brown, 2004).

There are three categories of inhaler devices available:

- Pressurised metered-dose inhalers (MDIs), e.g. Evohaler®
- Breath-actuated inhalers (BAIs), e.g. Autohaler® and Easi-Breath®
- Dry powder inhalers (DPIs), e.g. Accuhaler®, Aerohaler®, Clickhaler®, Diskhaler®, HandiHaler®, Turbohaler®

Pressurised Metered-Dose Inhalers

The pressurised metered-dose inhaler (MDI) is the most commonly used inhaler device (Figure 6.1). However, these require a degree of manual dexterity and good 'hand–breath' coordination to deliver the drug correctly, which may be difficult for frail and elderly patients with COPD. The drug, which is either dissolved or suspended in a propellant under pressure, is manually actuated and delivered at a rate of about 70 mph (Booker, 2004a).

Table 6.3. Advantages and disadvantages of inhaler devices

Device	Advantages	Disadvantages
MDI	Generic formulations available Inexpensive Compatible with spacer device Dose counter available on some inhalers	Hand–breath coordination required Requires reasonable amount of dexterity
Easi-Breath®	Easy to use	No dose counter
Autohaler®	Requires no coordination	On inhalation, click may put some patients off
Turbohaler®	Little or no taste Easy to use Last 20 doses indicator Dose counter on some Requires no coordination	More expensive than MDI Adequate inspirational effort required Requires reasonable amount of dexterity
Accuhaler®	Easy to use Requires no coordination Dose counter Last 5 doses indicator	More expensive than MDI Adequate inspirational effort required Requires reasonable amount of dexterity Compound rather gritty
Diskhaler®	Dose counter Requires no coordination	More expensive than MDI Fiddly to load Requires refills Compound rather gritty
Clickhaler®	Easy to use Last 10 doses indicator Requires no coordination Lock-out when empty	More expensive than MDI
Aerohaler®	Easy to use Requires no coordination	No dose counter On inhalation, click may put some patients off
HandiHaler®	Dose can be monitored Requires no coordination Little or no taste	Device rather stiff when new Fiddly to load More expensive than MDI Requires reasonable amount of dexterity

Therefore, a good inhaler technique is vital to prevent it being deposited in the mouth or back of the throat and swallowed. Even with a good inhaler technique the drug deposition in the lungs from an MDI is less than 20% of the dose, the majority being deposited in the oropharynx (Benson and Prankered, 1998). Frequent inhaler technique checks are important as it is

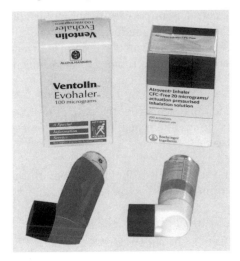

Figure 6.1. Pressurised metered-dose inhalers (MDIs)

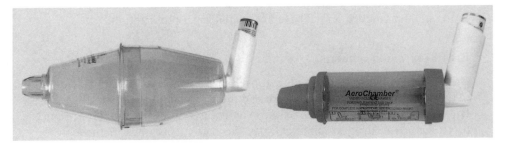

Figure 6.2. Volumatic® and AeroChamber® device

reported that 75% of patients with COPD are unable to use them correctly (Connolly, 1995).

One method of overcoming coordination problems with MDIs is to use them with a spacer device (Figure 6.2). There are several available and it is important that the spacer and MDI are compatible. Spacer devices are more effective and increase the amount of drug deposition in the lungs and reduce the side effects in the mouth and throat, particularly in the case of inhaled steroids. Used correctly high doses from a hand-held inhaler and spacer will usually produce the same effect as nebulised bronchodilators (Jenkins, Heaton and Fulton, 1987). The main disadvantage is that the Volumatic® is bulky and not very portable, although the Ablespacer® and Aerochamber® are slightly smaller.

When using a spacer, it is important to inhale as soon as possible after activating the MDI as the drug remains in the aerosol form for only a short time. Only one puff should be activated at a time, with a gap of 30–60 seconds between puffs. There are two methods for breathing the drug through a spacer:

• After activating the inhaler instruct the patient to take one deep breath in and hold for 5–10 seconds and repeat the process for a second dose, shaking the inhaler in between.

For patients who find it difficult to hold their breath the following method known as 'tidal breathing' would be more suitable:

• After activating the inhaler instruct the patient to hold the spacer to their lips and breath in and out slowly and gently four or five times for each puff, repeating the process for a second dose, shaking the inhaler in between.

For patients who are able to use an MDI but have problems activating the dose due to arthritis, a Haleraid® 200 is available which can easily be fitted to the inhaler (Figure 6.3). These are available on prescription.

Breath-Actuated Inhalers

Breath-actuated inhalers provide a convenient, portable and effective method of delivering drug therapy and overcome the coordination problems of MDIs. Breath-actuated inhalers such as the Autohaler® and Easi-Breath® (Figure 6.4) release the drug automatically as the patient breathes in through the mouthpiece, therefore removing the need to press and breathe at the same time. The main disadvantage of the breath-actuated inhaler is that some patients may stop inhaling when the inhaler 'fires'.

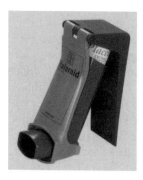

Figure 6.3. Haleraid®

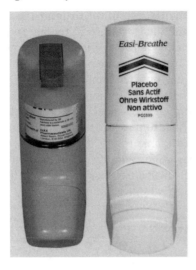

Figure 6.4. Breath-actuated inhalers (BAIs)

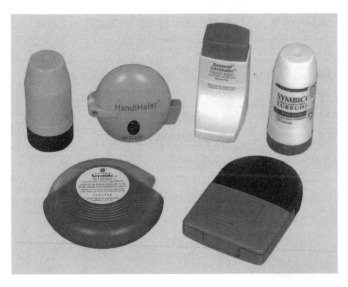

Figure 6.5. Selection of dry powder inhalers (DPIs) available

Dry Powder Inhalers

A variety of dry powder inhalers (DPIs) are available to choose from (Figure 6.5) and do not require hand–breath coordination to activate. To be effective, however, they do require a sufficient inspirational flow of 30–90 L/min, depending on the device to carry the drug powder from the inhaler into the lungs. Used correctly the deposition of drug in the lungs is approximately 30% of the dose (Brown, 2004). Although more expensive, Allen and Prior (1986) report that around 90% of patients use dry powder inhalers correctly, making them more cost effective.

To assess whether a dry powder inhaler would be suitable for patients or whether they have adequate inspirational effort their inspiratory flow rate can be measured using an 'In-check Dial®' made by Clement Clarke (Figure 6.6). Symbicort® also produce a placebo whistle trainer (Figure 6.7) to ensure that patients are able to use it correctly before prescribing. These are available from drug representatives. For patients who are able to use Symbicort® but have problems twisting the inhaler to activate the dose due

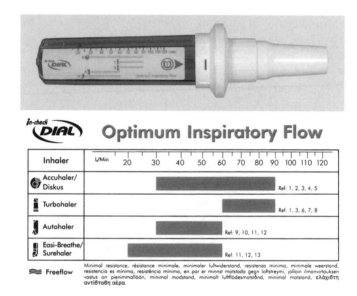

Figure 6.6. 'In-check Dial®' and chart. Reproduced by permission of Clement Clarke

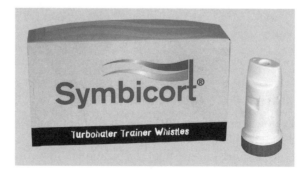

Figure 6.7. Symbicort® whistle trainer

to arthritis and difficulty in grasping, a turning aid is available which can be fitted on to the bottom of the Turbohaler® (Figure 6.8). These are available from drug representatives.

NEBULISER THERAPY

A nebuliser is a device that converts a drug solution into a fine aerosol of appropriate particle size of 1–5 μm to penetrate the small airways in order to produce optimal effect (Higenbottam, 1997). The nebuliser compressor (Figure 6.9) drives the nebuliser by drawing the drug solution within the nebuliser by fragmenting it into particles. The fine aerosol mist is then inhaled by the patient breathing normally over a 5–10 minute period until the solution has dispersed. A mouthpiece is usually used by the patient to deliver the nebulised solution rather than a facemask, owing to the small risk of precipitating glaucoma when ipratropium bromide is used via a facemask. The most commonly used domiciliary nebuliser is the standard jet nebuliser, which should comply with European standards drawn up by the European Committee for Standardisation. Compressors should be serviced yearly along with an electrical safety check. Nebuliser equipment (i.e. chamber and mask/mouthpiece) should be washed in warm soapy water and dried thoroughly after each use and stored in a plastic bag to keep it clean and dust free. Patients should be instructed to replace these according to the manufacturer's instructions, which is usually 3 monthly. NICE guidelines (National Collaborating Centre for Chronic Conditions, 2004) recommend that if a nebuliser is prescribed for a patient they should be provided with the equipment, servicing, advice and support.

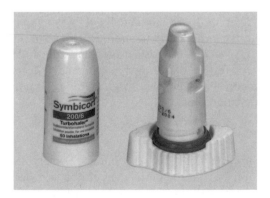

Figure 6.8.   Turning aid for the Symbicort Turbohaler®

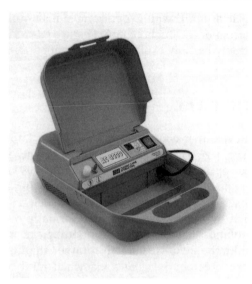

Figure 6.9.   Nebuliser compressor. Reproduced by permission of Clement Clarke

Indications for Nebuliser Therapy

The British Thoracic Society (1997a) has published detailed guidelines on the use of nebuliser therapy and recommend that patients are receiving optimal treatment prior to being assessed for a nebuliser. Nebuliser therapy may be considered for patients at home with COPD for a number of reasons:

- Patients who no longer find inhalers effective
- Patients who require large doses of inhaled drugs to control their symptoms of breathlessness
- During an acute exacerbation of COPD
- Patients who have become too frail or ill to use inhalers effectively

Although high doses of drugs can be delivered via a nebuliser it is a costly and a time-consuming process. Patients may also experience more severe systemic side effects from the drugs, such as tachycardia and tremor. However, patients with distressing or disabling breathlessness despite using inhaler therapy should be considered for nebuliser therapy (National Collaborating Centre for Chronic Conditions, 2004).

Nebuliser Trials

The BTS Nebuliser Guidelines (British Thoracic Society, 1997a) recommend that prior to a nebuliser trial the patient should be assessed using high-dose bronchodilator therapy with up to 6–8 puffs four hourly via a spacer device.

A hospital specialist or a GP with experience of nebuliser trials may carry out a nebuliser assessment. Details of how to use and care for the nebuliser and compressor should be fully explained to the patient, noting that the trial is likely to last 4–8 weeks as follows:

- Weeks 1–2: administer 6–8 puffs of high-dose bronchodilator therapy via a spacer device.
- Weeks 3–4: administer short-acting bronchodilator via a nebuliser (e.g. salbutamol 2.5–5 mg or terbutaline 5–10 mg four times a day).
- Weeks 5–6: administer anticholinergic only (e.g. ipratropium bromide 250–500 µg four times a day).
- Weeks 7–8: combine short-acting bronchodilator and anticholinergic in a nebuliser four times a day.

The patient should be assessed and nebuliser therapy continued only if one or more of the following is confirmed (National Collaborating Centre for Chronic Conditions, 2004):

- A reduction in symptoms
- An increase in the ability to undertake various activities of living, which the patient was not able to do before
- An increase in exercise capacity
- An improvement in lung function

It is important to remember that nebulised bronchodilator therapy may lead to significant improvements in symptoms, exercise capacity or quality of life, which are not reflected in changes in FEV_1. Although nebuliser therapy is a basic treatment in the management of COPD the availability of a nebuliser service varies throughout the UK.

MISCELLANEOUS COPD THERAPY

Influenza Vaccination

Since 1993, the Department of Health has recommended that all patients with COPD, especially the elderly at risk, receive an annual influenza vaccination. Although no specific trials have been conducted regarding the efficacy of vaccination of patients with chronic respiratory disease, specifically in COPD against influenza, there is evidence to suggest a reduction in acute admissions and death rates from influenza (Gorse *et al.*, 1997).

Pneumococcus Vaccination

Streptococcus pneumoniae is the most common cause of community-acquired pneumonia (Bellamy and Booker, 2003). Polyvalent pneumococcal vaccine is used to protect against the development of pneumococcal infections, usually as a single lifetime injection. However, immunocompromised patients or patients having had a splenectomy are usually given booster injections every five years. This has been shown to reduce the incidence of invasive pneumococcal infection in patients with chronic lung disease and to be cost effective (Hansel and Barnes, 2004). A study by Nichol *et al.* (1999) over two influenza seasons looked at a cohort ($n = 1989$) of elderly people with chronic lung disease given only pneumococcal vaccination. The findings demonstrated a reduction in the number of hospitalisations (43%) for pneumonia and influenza, and a reduction in the risk of death (29%) from all causes. A further study by Nichol *et al.* (1999) looked at the benefits over three influenza seasons of both influenza and pneumococcal vaccinations among a cohort ($n = 1898$) of elderly people with chronic lung disease. The results indicated a reduction (63%) in the risk for hospitalisation with pneumonia and a reduction (81%) in the risk of death versus when neither vaccination had been received.

MUCOLYTIC THERAPY

Until very recently mucolytic therapy has not been available within the UK, although it has been widely available in Europe. This has been due to the lack of evidence on their effectiveness in COPD, particularly in those patients with an FEV_1 of <50% predicted. However, NICE guidelines (National Collaborating Centre for Chronic Conditions, 2004) recommend the use of mucolytic therapy in patients with a chronic productive cough, which can be particularly troublesome and embarrassing for some patients. The aim of treatment is to thin the secretions, making them easier to expectorate, and therefore to reduce the frequency of the cough. Studies by Poole and Black (2001) have shown that mucolytic therapy can also reduce the number of exacerbations in some patients.

Currently the only mucolytic agent that can be prescribed in the UK is carbocysteine (Mucodyne®). It is recommended that it should be tried in patients with a chronic productive cough for one month and continued if there is a clear clinical benefit. Patients should also be encouraged to drink plenty of water if this is a particular problem, to help keep sputum thin and easy to expectorate (Esmond, 2001).

PROPHYLACTIC ANTIBIOTIC THERAPY

Prophylactic antibiotic therapy has been used in the past in an attempt to prevent exacerbations in patients with COPD. However, with the few studies that have been conducted there remains insufficient evidence to recommend prophylactic antibiotic therapy as appropriate in the management of COPD. Most of the studies lacked standardisation, which showed systematic bias and considered only small sample sizes (National Collaborating Centre for Chronic Conditions, 2004).

SHORT-BURST OXYGEN THERAPY

Short-burst oxygen therapy is commonly prescribed within the community and is one of the most expensive therapies used in the NHS. Patients with COPD often use short-burst oxygen therapy when experiencing excessive breathlessness following exertion, and cannot get relief using other treatments. Some patients with severe COPD may experience a fall in their oxygen saturations post-exertion and take some time to recover. Short-burst oxygen therapy can help them to recover quicker and help relieve their breathlessness. Previous studies have shown variable results on the use of short-burst oxygen therapy, providing mainly subjective evidence of its value. In particular, Woodcock, Grodd and Geddes (1981) demonstrated some improvement in exercise capacity and dyspnoea when using short-burst oxygen therapy before exercise, but oxygen saturations were not measured.

Although some patients do appear to benefit from short-burst oxygen therapy, especially those that do not meet the criteria for long-term oxygen therapy, it is important that all other treatments are tried, including breathing control exercises, before oxygen cylinders are introduced. Patients can easily become over-reliant on the use of oxygen, which may simply have a placebo effect due to the feeling of cool air on the face rather than a true therapeutic effect, i.e. correction of hypoxia.

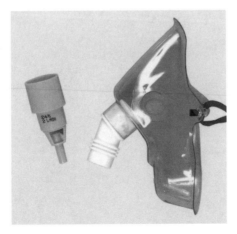

Figure 6.10.   Oxygen face mask and 24% venturi

Patients using oxygen for intermittent relief post-exertion should have an oxygen mask (with a 24% venturi) (Figure 6.10) attached to the cylinder rather than nasal cannulae. This is because very often these patients will be mouth-breathing and will gain more benefit from the use of a facemask. Patients should be instructed to turn the oxygen cylinder on to medium flow (2 L/min) and use the oxygen for short bursts of 5–10 minutes at a time and then to turn the oxygen off. The number of cylinders used by each patient should be documented.

Chapter 7

Management of Acute Exacerbations of COPD

INTRODUCTION

Exacerbations are significant events for patients with COPD. As the severity of COPD progresses, so the number of exacerbations usually increases. These events are not only distressing and disruptive to the patient, affecting their quality of life and daily activities, but also account for a high proportion of the total health costs of caring for patients with COPD (National Collaborating Centre for Chronic Conditions, 2004). Many patients with mild to moderate exacerbations of COPD will be managed appropriately in the community by their GP and specialist nurse/physiotherapist. Patients with severe COPD are usually more prone to developing further complications as a result of their exacerbation and often need medical treatment and admission to secondary care.

DEFINITION OF AN EXACERBATION

Although exacerbations of COPD are fairly common there appears to be no widely accepted definition of an acute exacerbation, partly due to the inherent difficulties of defining exacerbation (Rodriguez-Roisin, 2000). However, NICE guidelines (National Collaborating Centre for Chronic Conditions, 2004) state the following:

> An exacerbation is a sustained worsening of the patient's symptoms from their usual state that is beyond normal day-to-day variations, with an acute onset. Additional treatment is required to treat any increase in symptoms.

The general symptoms of an exacerbation include:

- Increasing breathlessness
- Cough

- Increased sputum production
- Increased sputum purulence

Mild exacerbations may present with one or two of the above symptoms while moderate exacerbations may present with two or three of the above. Other symptoms may include upper respiratory symptoms such as a cold or sore throat, increased wheeze and chest tightness, reduced exercise tolerance, fatigue and general malaise.

A severe exacerbation will present with all the above symptoms including some or all of the following:

- Tachypnea and tachycardia
- Pyrexia
- Use of accessory muscles (sternomastoid and abdominal) of respiration at rest
- Pursed-lip breathing
- Central cyanosis
- Reduced alertness or confusion
- Evidence of right heart failure and peripheral oedema
- Marked reduction in ability to perform daily activities of living
- Reduce spirometry
- Reduced oxygen saturations

CAUSES OF AN EXACERBATION

The most common causes of an exacerbation of COPD are either viral or bacterial infections, particularly during the winter months. Pathogens responsible are usually *Haemophilus influenzae, Streptococcus pneumoniae, Moraxella catarrhalis* and *Chlamydia pneumoniae* (Wedzicha, 2002). However, a third of exacerbations have no obvious cause or signs of infection. The cause may relate to a change in temperature, weather conditions or increased pollutant factors. Very often, on these occasions lung function may remain unchanged.

It is important to always bear in mind that increasing or worsening symptoms may be caused by other conditions, which should be considered and excluded when making a diagnosis of an exacerbation (National Collaborating Centre for Chronic Conditions, 2004):

- Pneumonia
- Pneumothorax
- Left ventricular failure or pulmonary oedema
- Pulmonary embolism
- Lung cancer

- Pleural effusion
- Upper airway obstruction

MANAGEMENT OF AN ACUTE EXACERBATION

Exacerbations of COPD in patients with mild to moderate disease are usually managed at home with appropriate antibiotics, and if required steroids, with a full recovery. Patients with severe COPD tend to have more frequent infections (more than 3 a year), take longer to recover and their lung function may not return to pre-exacerbation level before a further exacerbation occurs. For these patients, frequent exacerbations often lead to a progressive deterioration of their condition, which may in some cases require admission to hospital. The decision whether to admit or not can sometimes be a difficult one to make. It is important that all factors are considered including medical and social factors. The NICE guidelines (National Collaborating Centre for Chronic Conditions, 2004) list the various factors to consider when deciding to treat an acute exacerbation at home or in hospital (Table 7.1). This involves the assessment of the severity of the patient's symptoms, in particular the degree of breathlessness at rest and when talking, how alert the patient is and the presence of cyanosis or peripheral oedema. The ability to perform daily activities, whether living alone or not, and the degree of mobility are also important factors to consider.

Table 7.1. Criteria for deciding whether to treat an acute exacerbation of COPD at home or in hospital. Taken from National Collaborating Centre for Chronic Conditions (2004)

Symptoms/factors	Treat at home	Refer/treat in hospital
Ability to cope at home	Yes	No
Breathlessness	Mild	Severe
General condition	Good	Poor/deteriorating
Level of activity	Good	Poor/confined to bed
Cyanosis	No	Yes
Worsening peripheral oedema	No	Yes
Level of consciousness	Alert	Impaired
Receiving long-term oxygen therapy (LTOT)	No	Yes
Social circumstances	Good	Living alone/not coping
Acute confusion	No	Yes
Rapid onset	No	Yes
Significant co-morbidity	No	Yes
Changes on chest X-ray	No	Yes
Arterial pH level	>7.35	<7.35
Arterial PaO$_2$	>7 kPa	<7 kPa

TREATMENT OF AN EXACERBATION AT HOME

Most patients with a mild or moderate exacerbation can be managed at home with appropriate treatment to relieve symptoms and to treat any infection present. In many areas of the UK the development of community nurse-led respiratory care teams who have specialist skills and knowledge in the management of COPD in the community have been established (Gravil *et al.*, 1999; Barnett, 2003). This additional service provides advice and support to GPs, patients and carers, avoiding where possible (and where it is safe to do so) admission to hospital. The roles of such teams of specialist nurses are to ensure that patients are receiving optimal treatment for their exacerbation, including nebuliser and oxygen therapy if required. Visits are usually made on a daily basis or as the patient's condition warrants, to monitor his or her condition and provide advice and support to both the patient and carers until fully recovered (Barnett, 2003). Patients and carers find this kind of service provision very comforting and beneficial to have their acute episodes managed at home by a visiting specialist nurse. From a GP's perspective, such services can have an impact on surgery time and ease the burden of frequent home visits during the day and out of hours.

Antibiotics

It is common practice to prescribe antibiotics for infective exacerbations of COPD if two or more of the following are present:

- Increasing breathlessness
- Increased sputum production
- Purulent sputum

Antibiotic choice will depend on local microbiology protocols, but in general amoxycillin (500 mg TDS), clarithromycin (500 mg BD) or trimethoprim (200 mg BD), usually for seven days, is adequate for most patients. Sputum culture is not usually indicated for these patients.

Oral Corticosteroids

Oral corticosteroids have been shown to improve recovery, spirometry and symptoms rapidly. Oral corticosteroids may be of benefit in exacerbations not caused by infection, where patients present with increased breathlessness and wheeze and reduced spirometry readings. They may also be added to anti-biotic therapy for an infective exacerbation accompanied by increased breathlessness and wheeze. A course of prednisolone 30 mg daily for 7 days is usually adequate. Patients on long-term maintenance oral steroids will require their dose increased to 30 mg, although some patients may require 40 mg daily, for

7 days and then reducing their dose over a couple of weeks back to their previous maintenance dose.

Bronchodilators

Prescribing a short-acting beta agonist (salbutamol, Ventolin®, Salamol®, Asmasal®) or anticholinergic (ipratropium bromide) bronchodilator can relieve symptoms of increased breathlessness if the patient is not already receiving this treatment. If already taking this treatment the dose of both inhalers should be increased to 4 hourly via a space device to increase drug deposition in the lungs. The patient's inhaler technique should be checked to ensure that the patient is using the inhalers correctly. Very occasionally a nebuliser may be required for an acute exacerbation, particularly if the patient has problems inhaling the medication due to increased breathlessness. On these occasions Combivent® nebules 4–6 hourly via a nebuliser are appropriate to use for 5 days until the patient is fully recovered and can then revert back to their inhalers. Usually a high dose of inhaled bronchodilator (4 puffs = 400 mg) via a space device can be just as effective if taken correctly.

Diuretics

The use of diuretic therapy is not routinely required in the management of acute exacerbations of COPD. However, patients who develop peripheral oedema may require a small dose of diuretic therapy to relieve the discomfort of the peripheral oedema. Care should be taken to monitor serum potassium levels, especially if the patient is receiving high-dose beta agonist therapy.

Nursing Interventions

In addition to the above course of treatments, patients should be encouraged to maintain an adequate fluid intake, in particular water, to reduce the stickiness of sputum and to help with expectorating. Light frequent meals should also be encouraged, particularly if they are very breathless or if their appetites have diminished. Patients should be advised to maintain a good posture, sitting upright well supported by pillows and to remain in bed for as little time as possible to prevent other complications occurring as a result of immobility. Patients should try and conserve energy to avoid getting too tired and breathless. If expectorating is a particular problem, deep breathing and huffing exercises should be encouraged 3–4 times daily and steam inhalations may be of benefit. If sputum retention is causing some distress a community physiotherapist may be required to assist with clearance of chest secretions. Patients may also find an electric fan of benefit when very breathless.

Follow-up

Patients treated with an exacerbation at home usually respond well to treatment and make a full recovery. They should also be advised regarding their usual optimal bronchodilator therapy and oral steroid therapy if on a maintenance dose. For some patients it may be advisable for them to keep an emergency stock of antibiotics and steroids at home with clear guidelines, so that they are able to initiate treatment without delay when required to prevent symptoms becoming too severe and requiring admission to hospital. Opportunities should never be missed to reiterate advice regarding smoking, diet and the importance of exercise and keeping active.

Patients who fail to respond to treatment and make a full recovery may require further examination and assessment to exclude other differential diagnosis. Investigations such as a chest X-ray, sputum cultures or referral to a respiratory specialist may be required.

MANAGEMENT OF AN EXACERBATION IN HOSPITAL

Acute exacerbations of COPD account for the second most common cause of medical admissions in the UK (Fehrenbach, 2005). The average district general hospital will receive between 1000 and 1200 admissions a year (Davis *et al.*, 2000; Barnett, 2003), with a mean stay of 10.3 days (Johnson and Stevenson, 2002). In return this has a major impact on hospital resources, which places increasing pressure on acute medical beds and on Accident and Emergency (A&E) services. In 2000, the cost to the NHS of caring for respiratory patients was estimated at £2.5 billion, with around two-fifths of these costs being for inpatient care (Respiratory Alliance, 2003). COPD patients, in particular, have a high incidence of readmission to hospital, with around 34% of patients being readmitted within a 3 month period (Roberts *et al.*, 2002). In addition, hospital mortality due to an acute exacerbation of COPD is approximately 10%, which exceeds the current hospital rates for myocardial infarction (Gravil *et al.*, 1999).

Patients with a severe exacerbation of COPD who are not responding to treatment or are generally deteriorating will require admission to hospital. Admission will also be necessary if the carers are unable to cope or if the patient is becoming very tired. Factors such as increased breathlessness, cyanosis, worsening ankle oedema and confusion can all indicate the development of complications and the need for hospital management.

Following admission, the main aims of management are to assess the severity of the patient's condition and to treat appropriately. A full history of onset, treatment and examination of the patient will be required. Clinical observations and oxygen saturations should be recorded. Many large hospitals now have teams of specialist respiratory nurses, and operate 'hospital at home' schemes (Davis *et al.*, 2000) or 'acute rapid assessment services' (ARAS) (Gordois and Gibbons, 2002). 'Hospital at home' schemes aim to facilitate early discharge of patients admitted with an exacerbation of COPD. Such schemes have reduced a patient's length of stay in hospital from 10 average bed days to less than 4 days, which provide support and a customized home treatment package provided by specialist nurses. Randomised controlled trials (Gravil *et al.*, 1999; Cotton *et al.*, 2000; Davis *et al.*, 2000) have demonstrated that such schemes are cost effective, safe, with no increase in morbidity or readmission rates, and were acceptable to patients who preferred to be home. Acute rapid assessment services identify those patients who can be safely managed at home with additional nursing and social input rather than being admitted to hospital.

Investigations

Patients admitted to hospital with an exacerbation of COPD will require the following tests (National Collaborating Centre for Chronic Conditions, 2004):

- Chest X-ray (to exclude other causes of increased breathlessness such as pneumothorax, pleural effusion)
- Arterial blood gases
- ECG (to exclude co-morbidities)
- Full blood count, urea and electrolytes
- Sputum microscopy and culture (if sputum is purulent)
- Blood cultures (if patient is pyrexial)
- Theophylline levels (if taking oral theophylline prior to admission)
- Record FEV_1 if the patient is able

Treatment

OXYGEN THERAPY

Many patients with a severe exacerbation of COPD may become significantly hypoxic and require controlled oxygen therapy. The amount administered will very much depend on the patient, but initially 24–28% via a venturi mask is given (Halpin, 2001) to ensure oxygen saturations do not fall below 90% (National Collaborating Centre for Chronic Conditions, 2004). However, it is not uncommon for patients to be transported to hospital via an ambulance having received high-flow oxygen and as a result are found to be hypercapnic or acidotic. NICE guidelines (National Collaborating Centre for Chronic Conditions, 2004) actually state that during transfer to hospital oxygen therapy should be commenced at 40% and titrated upwards only if saturations fall below 90% and should be reduced if saturations exceed 93–94% or if the patient becomes drowsy. Once in hospital arterial blood gas measurements should be repeated regularly until the patient has responded to treatment and is stabilised. Patients with pH < 7.35 or worsening hypercapnia may require noninvasive ventilation or admission to intensive care, if appropriate, until improved.

DRUG THERAPY

Bronchodilator therapy via a nebuliser of salbutamol (2.5–5 mg) and ipratropium bromide (500 µg) 6 hourly is the mainstay of patients admitted with a severe exacerbation of COPD. If ineffective, intravenous aminophylline (500 µg/kg h) may also be required to help stabilise the patient. Caution is needed when using intravenous aminophylline because of the interactions with other drugs and potential toxicity if the patient has been prescribed oral theophylline prior to admission.

Oral corticosteroids are administered in conjunction with other therapies for patients admitted to hospital with an exacerbation of COPD. The recommended dose is 30 mg orally initially for 5–7 days. Antibiotic therapy will also be required, especially if the sputum is purulent or there is evidence on the patient's chest X-ray confirming pneumonia. Initially antibiotic treatment is given orally and should be an aminopenicillin, a macrolide or a tetracycline, depending on guidance issued by local microbiologists. Sputum sent for culture should be treated accordingly against culture and sensitivity when made available.

RESPIRATORY STIMULANTS

During severe exacerbations of COPD some patients may develop hypercapnic ventilatory failure, which is usually managed using noninvasive ventilation within the respiratory ward setting. However, if noninvasive ventilation is either not available or considered inappropriate for the patient, especially if the patient is drowsy or comatose, it is recommended that doxapram is used. Doxapram is a respiratory stimulant administered intravenously via injection or infusion and has a short duration of action. In the short term it may stabilise the patient sufficiently to enable him or her to cooperate using noninvasive ventilation and to clear secretions if present. During administration the patient will require careful monitoring attached to a cardiac monitor and pulse oximeter as well as regular observations and frequent arterial blood gas measurements. Side effects include an increase in blood pressure, tachycardia, bradycardia, extrasystoles, dyspnoea, confusion, hallucinations and vomiting (British National Formulary, 2005).

DISCHARGE PLANNING FROM HOSPITAL

Discharge planning provides the opportunity for nursing and medical staff to assess the patient's medical and social needs prior to discharge back home into the community. Early COPD discharge schemes can provide support and advice and facilitate the patient's discharge home. A thorough and well-planned discharge will not only reduce the likelihood of the patient being readmitted, but also assist the multidisciplinary teams in the management of the patient once home. Communication between the patient, carers, family, GP and multidisciplinary teams involved in the patient's care is key to a successful discharge back into the community. Any social problems should be identified early during the admission to enable the appropriate agencies to conduct a full assessment and implement additional help and support as required.

Once the patient is responding well to medical treatment this should be reviewed by COPD specialist teams to facilitate early discharge home. Patients commenced on nebulised therapy for an acute exacerbation will need to be transferred back on to their usual inhaled therapy at least 24 hours prior to their discharge from hospital, or sooner if possible. This provides adequate opportunity to assess the patient's inhaler technique and provide further education concerning the correct use of all the medication. Where possible every opportunity should be taken to document the patient's list of medication to prevent any confusion when the patient is at home.

Patients who have required oxygen therapy during their treatment will need to be assessed daily and oxygen saturations measured, which should be weaned appropriately. Once patients have stabilised, oxygen therapy should be discontinued to prevent the patient becoming over-reliant on it. Patients who usually receive oxygen at home should also be weaned to their usual treatment. Patients who were admitted with respiratory failure may require arterial blood gas analysis prior to discharge to ensure these are satisfactory.

Prior to discharge, spirometry should be measured if possible and arrangements should be made for the COPD team to follow up at home and provide support and advice to the patient and family. Such teams can also provide appropriate health education tailored to the patient's individual needs and the various stages of each patient's disease.

SELF-MANAGEMENT EDUCATION

Self-management education and action plans have been successfully used for some time for patients with asthma. These patients are encouraged to record their peak flow if they detect any variations in symptoms and lung function. If their peak flow falls below a specific reading, patients are instructed to take appropriate action regarding their medication. Unfortunately, peak expiratory flow readings are rarely useful in COPD and as yet there is no simple device for patients to monitor their FEV$_1$. To date, there has been very little research or evidence published to suggest that self-management education/ plans would be as effective in the management of exacerbations in COPD, although the NICE guidelines (National Collaborating Centre for Chronic Conditions, 2004) support the need for further studies. However, supportive interventions, directed at helping patients manage their chronic disease rather than their disease controlling them, are likely to increase their confidence in managing their condition rather than encouraging dependency on others.

The main aim of self-management is to educate the patient in recognising the early signs of an exacerbation so that prompt action can be taken to

Table 7.2. COPD self-management education plan

Lifestyle change suggestions
1. Stop smoking/discuss smoking cessation
2. Keep active and take daily exercise. Remember getting breathless is not harmful. Undertake pulmonary rehabilitation programme if possible
3. Learn to adjust daily activities of living and conserve energy
4. Use effective breathing control exercises
5. Eat a balanced diet little and often. Include plenty of fresh fruit and vegetables. Drink plenty of fluids, in particular water
6. Wrap up warm in cold weather
7. Ensure yearly flu vaccination and Pneumovax

Usual spirometry readings:
FEV$_1$: .... FVC: .... FEV$_1$/FVC %: .... PEF: ....
Oxygen saturations on air: ....On oxygen ....litres: ....

Medication options for worsening symptoms
Reliever:
Take extra .... inhaler/nebuliser up to ....
....

Signs of a chest infection:
If you notice two or more of the following:
• Increasingly short of breath
• Increased amount of sputum
• Sputum has changed colour and green
you are advised to start your 'emergency supply' of antibiotics and steroids

Antibiotics:
Take ....mg(.................tabs)
..............times a day for ....days

Steroids (prednisolone):
Take ....mg(.................tabs)
..............times a day for ....days

If your condition does not improve or your condition deteriorates please ensure your either contact your GP or respiratory nurse.

prevent their condition becoming worse and needing admission. Patients can hold an 'emergency stock', thereby responding promptly to the symptoms of an exacerbation by starting oral corticosteroid therapy if their breathlessness interferes with activities of living, and starting antibiotic therapy if their sputum is purulent as well as adjusting their bronchodilator therapy to control their symptoms (National Collaborating Centre for Chronic Conditions, 2004). Patients should have a clear understanding that they should inform their respiratory nurse or GP when they have started such treatment so that this can be recorded and also to ensure that they recover fully from the exacerbation. If at any time their condition does not improve or deteriorates, clear instructions should be given to the patient to contact their respiratory nurse or GP.

Self-management education and plans should include both lifestyle advice and advice regarding self-medication if they develop symptoms of an exacerbation (Table 7.2). This information is best provided both written and verbally so that the patient has something to refer to. Documenting the patient's usual spirometry and oximetry readings within the plan is also useful, particularly for other health care professionals visiting the home or if the patient is admitted to A&E in an emergency. Realistic goals and expectations are an important part of self-management and if tailored to individual needs can enhance a patient's quality of life and improve symptom control, and in the long term reduce hospital admissions. However, further studies are needed to establish if this is the case.

Chapter 8

Other Treatments in the Management of COPD

INTRODUCTION

There is no curative treatment for COPD. Therefore the management of the disease is directed at symptom control and improvement in functional status over and above that achieved by optimal medical treatment (American Thoracic Society, 1999). This chapter considers other specialist treatments available to patients with COPD other than smoking cessation and pharmacology.

Pulmonary rehabilitation is a multidisciplinary and holistic approach to patient care. The elements of such a programme focus on various aspects such as exercise and health education to improve the patient's quality of life and exercise tolerance.

Long-term oxygen therapy of at least 15 hours per day has been shown to improve the survival of patients with severe COPD. Noninvasive positive pressure ventilation (NIPPV) is a treatment commonly used on respiratory wards in the management of patients admitted with acute respiratory failure during exacerbations of COPD. Such treatment is now used as an alternative to invasive mechanical ventilation.

An alternative to medical intervention is the option of lung surgery. Such surgical procedures as bullectomy, lung volume reduction surgery (LVRS) and lung transplantation are now available to treat patients with COPD. A detailed individual assessment is required to assess the surgical risk factors involved in relation to the potential benefits including quality of life and survival of undergoing such a procedure.

PULMONARY REHABILITATION

In the past, the management of patients with COPD has very much focused on interventions either to prevent further deterioration in lung function such as smoking cessation or to improve lung function with the use of pharmacology. However, it is now evident that if patients can be taught and provided with specific knowledge regarding their condition, they are able to take control of their symptoms rather than the symptoms controlling them. The emphasis of pulmonary rehabilitation is therefore placed on reducing the disability associated with a chronic respiratory disease such as COPD.

Pulmonary rehabilitation involves a multidisciplinary approach incorporating the skills and knowledge from a wide range of health professionals. This usually includes a nurse, physiotherapist, occupational therapist, dietician, psychologist or counsellor and a benefits officer. Pulmonary rehabilitation is a programme that is individually tailored and designed to optimise each patient's physical performance and psychological wellbeing. Such programmes are becoming increasingly popular and an effective option in the management of patients with moderate to severe COPD. The benefits of such programmes include improvements in exercise performance, health-related quality of life, reduced breathlessness and reduction in the number of hospital admissions and GP visits (Lacasse *et al.*, 1996). As a consequence, this has an impact by reducing the usage of health services, making the programme effective and cost effective.

Traditionally, pulmonary rehabilitation programmes have been hospital based, usually on an outpatient basis. Recently community programmes have also been set up. These have a distinct advantage as they are usually easier to access and travelling time is reduced. To ensure a good attendance the right venue is important to run such programmes, bearing in mind the location, access and parking facilities. However, there are moves to develop home-based pulmonary rehabilitation programmes for patients who are housebound. Although these patients would miss out on the sharing of experiences of living with their condition, it is thought that such a programme in the home would be just as effective. Further research needs to be conducted within this area to assess the effectiveness of such programmes in the home regarding cost effectiveness and the impact on the patient's quality of life.

Programme Content

The British Thoracic Society (BTS) pulmonary rehabilitation guidelines state that programmes should run two sessions per week for a period of 6–8 weeks. However, 33% of the pulmonary rehabilitation programmes in the UK provided only one session a week (British Lung Foundation and British Thoracic Society, 2003). The aim of rehabilitation is broadly to restore the individual to the best possible level of physical and mental functioning (Morgan, 1999) by improving the patient's health and quality of life.

The content of the programme consists of an exercise component to increase endurance and muscle strengthening exercises. This involves gentle aerobic exercises including walking, step-ups, static bikes and climbing stars (Figure 8.1). The patient is required to carry out an individually tailored exercise programme at home in between sessions to increase their exercise tolerance.

The idea of starting an exercise programme may be rather daunting for patients with COPD. However, it must be emphasised to patients that breathlessness, although distressing, is not harmful and that keeping physically active is really important. The second component consists of education, providing information about the disease, its management and how to develop strategies in daily activities of living. The main topics covered include:

- The disease process
- Drug therapy
- Smoking cessation
- Symptom control
- Energy conservation
- Anxiety and relaxation technicians
- Nutrition
- Management of exacerbations
- Relationships
- Benefits advice
- Travel and holiday advice
- End-of-life decision making

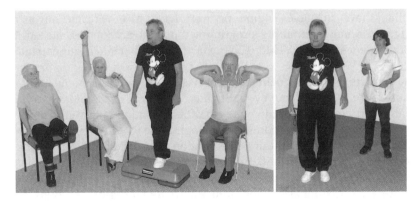

Figure 8.1. Pulmonary rehabilitation group and a patient performing a shuttle walk

Most programmes encourage carers to attend with the patient and can be invaluable in reinforcing the information learnt when the patient is at home and carrying out day-to-day activities.

Patient Selection

Patients with a diagnosis of moderate to severe COPD experiencing difficulties with exercise tolerance and daily activities as a result of breathlessness are generally included in pulmonary rehabilitation programmes. Indeed, the NICE guidelines (National Collaborating Centre for Chronic Conditions, 2004) recommend that pulmonary rehabilitation should be available to all patients who feel they are limited by their breathlessness (usually MRC grade 3 and above). However, patients should have a clear understanding of what the programme involves and that a degree of commitment is required on their part to obtain maximum benefit from the programme. Before a patient can participate in such a programme a baseline assessment is generally performed to assess suitability and to identify specific areas of improvement for individual patients. A patient should also be receiving optimal treatment.

The assessment involves:

- Confirmed diagnosis of COPD
- Recent chest X-ray, ECG and a full blood count to rule out any other causes of breathlessness
- Spirometry (before and after bronchodilator therapy)
- Assessment of exercise capacity with oximetry
- Measurement of health status (using questionnaires)
- Assessment of respiratory and general muscle strength

Pulmonary rehabilitation is not recommended for patients who have limited mobility, have unstable angina or who have had a recent myocardial infarction. Some community programmes do not accept patients on long-term oxygen therapy (LTOT) if hypoxia is a problem when the patient is at rest.

Despite its proven benefits, the provision of pulmonary rehabilitation remains poor. A recent survey highlighted that 10% of the pulmonary rehabilitation programmes running had no official funding and were run by the goodwill of staff and incorporated the programme within their existing workload and budget (British Lung Foundation and British Thoracic Society, 2003). The NICE COPD guidelines recommend that rehabilitation should be made available to all suitable patients who feel that they are functionally disabled by COPD (National Collaborating Centre for Chronic Conditions, 2004). Hopefully for the future this will provide the stimulus to improve the provision of such programmes for patients with COPD.

LONG-TERM OXYGEN THERAPY

Long-term oxygen therapy (LTOT) is used in patients with severe COPD and who become hypoxaemic. The aim of LTOT is to improve the quality of life and increase survival. Many patients tolerate mild hypoxaemia fairly well, but once the resting PaO_2 falls below 8 kPa patients may begin to develop signs of cor pulmonale. Once this occurs the prognosis is poor and if left untreated the 5 year survival rate of these patients is less than 50% (Halpin, 2001). Studies have shown that LTOT used for at least 15 hours per day not only increases survival but also reduced polycythaemia and progression of pulmonary hypertension, and showed some improvement in health status (Bellamy and Booker, 2003) (Table 8.1).

Domiciliary Oxygen Concentrators

Domiciliary oxygen concentrators have been available on the Drug Tariff since 1985. In 1999 around 18 000 concentrators were prescribed in the UK at an approximate cost of £683 rental per machine (Thompson, 2002). At present in England and Wales the patient's GP prescribes a concentrator, usually at the request of a respiratory physician following an assessment. However, from October 2005 new guidance has been issued from the Department of Health (2004a) to modernise the domiciliary oxygen service to improve access and to reduce the number of patients who receive the treatment inappropriately (Godfrey, 2004). The responsibility for ordering oxygen for LTOT will transfer from GPs to specialist consultants in secondary care. This hopefully will reduce the number of patients incorrectly prescribed LTOT, which not only restricts a patient's quality of life but also has no added benefit. It is also extremely expensive for the NHS (Godfrey, 2004).

Long-term oxygen therapy is delivered via an oxygen concentrator (Figure 8.2), which draws room air in through a series of filters to remove dust particles from the air. This air is then forced through two molecular sieve beds filled with a substance called zeolite. Here nitrogen and carbon dioxide are removed. The oxygen is then directed via a compressor through a flowmeter, which is regulated to the desired flow rate (McLauchlan, 2002). The concentrator runs off electricity, of which every quarter the cost is reimbursed to the

Table 8.1. Benefits of long-term oxygen therapy

Increased quality of life
Improved long-term survival
Prevention of deterioration in pulmonary hypertension
Reduction of polycythaemia
Improved quality of sleep
Reduction in cardiac arrhythmias

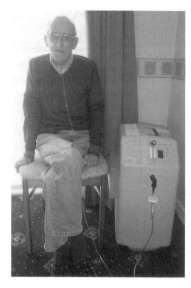

Figure 8.2. Patient using an oxygen concentrator in the home

patient. Oxygen tubing of up to 15 metres can be attached to the machine, which enables the patient to move around the home to aid mobility if required. It is an efficient, cost-effective and compact way of delivering oxygen and saves considerable storage space compared with oxygen cylinders. A back-up cylinder is always supplied in case of machine or power failure. The cost of supplying 15 hours of oxygen per day via size F oxygen cylinders would be around £6500 per year. In comparison the cost of a concentrator is considerably less at £1500 per year (Bellamy and Booker, 2003).

Indications for LTOT

Department of Health guidelines recommend that arterial blood gas measurements are made when the patient is clinically stable, on optimal therapy and measured on two occasions at least three weeks apart (Department of Health, 1999). In the 1980s two large multicentre trials demonstrated that long-term oxygen administered for 15 hours daily prolonged survival by approximate 30% in patients with severe COPD (Nocturnal Oxygen Therapy Trial, 1980; Medical Research Council, 1981). However, Lacasse *et al.* (1996) demonstrated in their study that long-term oxygen therapy does not improve survival in patients with mild to moderate hypoxaemia. The NICE COPD guidelines (National Collaborating Centre for Chronic Conditions, 2004) indicate that all patients with severe airflow obstruction ($FEV_1 < 30\%$ predicted) or cyanosis, raised jugular venous pressure or oxygen saturations <92% on air should be assessed for oxygen therapy (Table 8.2).

Table 8.2. Indicators for referral for LTOT assessment. Taken from National Collaborating Centre for Chronic Conditions (2004)

Severe COPD (FEV_1 < 30% predicted)
Patients with evidence of hypoxia (SaO_2 < 92%)
Polycythaemia
Cyanosis
Peripheral oedema
Raised jugular venous pressure
Right heart failure
Documented arterial blood gases PaO_2 < 7.3 kPa

The criteria for long-term oxygen therapy is indicated in patients with COPD who have a PaO_2 of less than 7.3 kPa when stable or a PaO_2 greater than 7.3 and less than 8 kPa when stable, with one of the following (National Collaborating Centre for Chronic Conditions, 2004):

• Peripheral oedema
• Pulmonary hypertension
• Secondary polycythaemia
• Nocturnal hypoxaemia (defined as SaO_2 below 90% for more than 30% of the night)

It is important that patients who meet the criteria requiring long-term oxygen therapy have stopped smoking. Evidence suggests that patients who continue to smoke gain no benefit from receiving LTOT (Bellamy and Booker, 2003), as well as being a safety hazard.

Methods of Oxygen Delivery

Long-term oxygen therapy is usually administered at a flow rate of 2, 3 or 4 litres per minute via nasal cannulae (Figure 8.3), as these are less cumbersome and less claustrophobic. They are also less obtrusive than a mask and enable the patient to carry out normal activities such as eating, drinking and talking without the need to remove them.

The oxygen is administered over a 15 hour period. This can be rather daunting for patients when this is initially discussed and they think that it will dominate their lives. However, it needs to be explained that the oxygen is administered over a period of time when they are usually resting. This is usually in the evening after their evening meal when they are watching television and during the night when asleep. This is usually at least 12 hours and then the remainder of the time is made up though the course of the day, usually in the afternoon if this is when they sit and relax for a further 3 hours to make a total of 15 hours. In this way patients do not need to let the oxygen therapy dominate their lives or feel tied to the house.

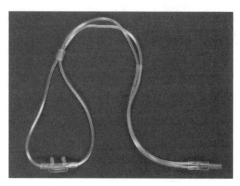

Figure 8.3. Nasal cannulae

Adverse effects are usually rare providing the patient has been assessed correctly and blood gas analysis completed on two separate occasions during a stable period. The most common flow rate of 2 litres of oxygen is prescribed and therefore the potential complication of progressive carbon dioxide retention is unlikely (Wegg and Hass, 1998).

Occasionally oxygen therapy can have a drying effect on the nasal mucosa, causing the nose to become sore and dry. Ensuring that the nasal prongs fit correctly and are not too long can prevent this. A water-based lubricating gel such as KY jelly (not soft white paraffin such as Vaseline as it is inflammable) may help and adequate fluids, in particular water, must be taken to avoid dehydration. It may be necessary to switch to a mask in the short term until the nose heals.

Another fairly common problem when initially using nasal cannulae is that the skin may become sore above the ears. This can be avoided by padding the tubing in these areas with foam to prevent friction.

Care and Management of Patients Using LTOT

Compliance with the use of LTOT has been found to be variable. Pepin (1996), in a prospective multicentred trial of 930 patients with COPD, found that only 419 patients used oxygen therapy effectively. On assessment patients should be fully informed of what LTOT involves and the commitment required by each individual patient in order for the therapy to be fully beneficial and effective. Therefore patient education via the respiratory nurse is an important aspect of prescribing LTOT, explaining exactly how and when to use the oxygen, how to apply the nasal cannulae and the occasional side effects that may occur.

The patient will require instructions on the care of the concentrator. It should be positioned in an area away from direct heat and where air can circulate sufficiently. It should also be placed out of reach of any children who may alter the flow rate or where it might get knocked accidentally. The machine should be wiped down with a damp cloth and the outside filter washed weekly in warm soapy water. A spare filter should be available to replace the one drying. The oxygen tubing should be checked regularly for kinks that may reduce the flow of oxygen and the nasal cannulae changed at least every three weeks (Matthews *et al.*, 2001). Health and safety issues should be outlined on the use of oxygen and reinforce the importance of nonsmoking by the patient and also family while the oxygen is in use.

Where possible the patient should be followed up at home by a respiratory nurse to check patient compliance and to identify potential problems or intolerance to treatment. Oxygen saturations should be recorded on air and oxygen to ensure these are stable. The new guidelines (Department of Health, 2004a) recommend that patients should receive support and six monthly visits and that patients are provided with contact details for the oxygen supplier and the visiting respiratory nurse.

If patients using LTOT are active, mobile and able to leave the house they may require ambulatory oxygen, especially if their oxygen saturations fall below 90% on a standard walking test, associated with an improvement in exercise tolerance or breathlessness (Royal College of Physicians, 1999). Portable oxygen cylinders, which are available on prescription, can have their limitations. They can be heavy for patients to handle and the short duration of gas supplied by them can limit patient activities (McLauchlan, 2002). The DD (Figure 8.4) and PA2 cylinders are lighter in weight than the PD

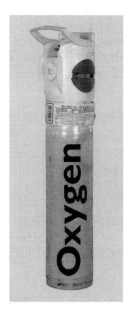

Figure 8.4. Portable DD oxygen cylinder

cylinder and provide a longer duration of gas of approximately 230 minutes. They also have the added advantage of an integral cylinder head, which reduced the need for exchanging cylinder heads. The PA2 also has the advantage of providing a wider range of flow rates from 0.5 to 15 litres per minute (McLauchlan, 2002).

The emphasis by health professionals to patients using LTOT is that the whole objective of using oxygen in the long term is to maximise their quality of life and exercise tolerance as well as improving their degree of breathlessness and survival rate in severe COPD.

Travel and Flying for Patients Using LTOT

Patients prescribed LTOT may still make arrangements to go away on holiday. Taking holidays in the UK is fairly straightforward and arrangements can be made to either transport the patient's own concentrator or make arrangements with the supplier to deliver one at the required destination. However, patients who wish to fly will often require advice regarding the need for supplementary oxygen during airline flights. It has been suggested that for patients to fly safely oxygen saturations should be greater than 92% on air and pre-flight PaO_2 should be more than 9.3 kPa with no evidence of hypercapnia. It is also not advisable for patients to fly with an FEV_1 of less than 25% predicted (Bellamy and Booker, 2003). This is due to the aircraft pressures, which are equivalent to 2438 m (8000 ft), reducing the partial pressure of oxygen to 15.1% oxygen at sea level (National Collaborating Centre for Chronic Conditions, 2004). In a healthy individual this will cause a significant drop from 12 to 8.7 kPa, which is equivalent to oxygen saturations of 96–90% (Bellamy and Booker, 2003). In patients with severe COPD this will exacerbate their levels of hypoxaemia unless they receive supplementary oxygen during the flight. The criteria for assessing the need for in-flight oxygen are shown in Table 8.3. COPD patients with large emphysematous bullae are at

Table 8.3. Assessing the need for in-flight oxygen. Taken from National Collaborating Centre for Chronic Conditions (2004)

Oxygen saturation	Oxygen requirement
$SaO_2 > 92\%$	Oxygen not required in flight
$SaO_2 > 92–95\%$ and no risk factors	Oxygen not required in flight
$SaO_2 > 92–95\%$: no additional risk factor including hypercapnia, ventilatory support, recent exacerbation, cardiac disease, cerebrovascular disease	Formal assessment of need for in-flight oxygen
	In-flight oxygen required
$SaO_2 < 92\%$: receiving supplementary oxygen	Increased flow rate while at cruising altitude

risk of developing a pneumothorax during flight due to the degree of volume expansion at reduced cabin pressure (National Collaborating Centre for Chronic Conditions, 2004). Travel by land or sea is not usually a problem for such patients.

The best advice for a patient is to be realistic when considering a holiday and plan in plenty of time. Many tour operators will help with arranging supplementary oxygen during the flight and a concentrator at the patient's destination. However, patients are advised to shop around as the cost can vary between airlines from a small fee up to £100. Most airlines require a GP letter confirming the patient's fitness to fly, while others will require a completed medical authorisation form. Patients can obtain further information on going on holiday from the British Lung Foundation. If there is any doubt about patients flying, they should be referred for further assessment by a respiratory physician. Some centres are able to conduct a hypoxic challenge by administering a reduced level of oxygen to assess their response during a flight.

NONINVASIVE VENTILATION

Noninvasive ventilation (NIV) is a method of providing ventilatory support that does not require the placement of an endotracheal tube and mechanical ventilation. It is a procedure that is commonly performed on a general respiratory ward or in an attached respiratory high-dependency unit rather than an intensive care unit. Over the last 10 years noninvasive ventilation has been a choice of treatment (Table 8.4) in the management of patients with acute hypercapnic respiratory failure (Type 2) following an exacerbation of COPD. Type 2 respiratory failure is defined as:

- pH < 7.35
- $PaO_2 < 7.5\,kPa$
- $PaCO_2 > 6.5\,kPa$

The main aim of using noninvasive ventilation acutely is to allow adequate oxygenation while relieving or preventing respiratory acidosis by increasing

Table 8.4. Clinical indications for the use of noninvasive ventilation

History of deteriorating blood gases (acidotic pH, hypoxaemia, hypercapnia)
Increased breathlessness
History of COPD

ventilation and removing $PaCO_2$. However, NIV is only suitable for patients providing they are able to cooperate and protect their own airways (Table 8.5). It would not be safe for patients with copious amounts of secretions or who are vomiting to use this form of treatment (Halpin, 2003).

Bilevel ventilators are commonly used that deliver two pressures: inspiratory positive airway pressure (IPAP) and expiratory positive airway pressure (EPAP). IPAP supports the breath, improves tidal volume, maximises the removal of carbon dioxide and reduces the work of breathing. EPAP acts as a splint and prevents the airways collapsing on expiration by reducing air-trapping and improving oxygenation, which in turn reduces the work of breathing (Riches, 2003). The two pressures are adjusted according to the patient's tolerance and response to treatment. This treatment is delivered via either a silicone face or a nasal mask (Figure 8.5). The nasal mask is less claustrophobic, but the patient must keep the mouth closed. If the patient is mouth-breathing a full-face mask is more appropriate. Most masks if fitted correctly do not require a dressing to the bridge of the nose to prevent a pressure ulcer developing. The ventilator is programmed to supplement the patient's own respiratory effort. If required, oxygen can be added to the circuit or to a valve on the mask.

Care and Management of Patients with NIV

Early identification of patients admitted with acute hypercapnic respiratory failure who may benefit from NIV depends on arterial blood gas analysis and the ability to maintain their own airways. Initially patients will require careful one-to-one nursing care and close monitoring by a competent trained nurse with the appropriate skills and knowledge. Patients will require support and encouragement to cooperate if they are to benefit from the treatment. The patient will require continuous pulse oximetry to monitor oxygen saturations (British Thoracic Society, 2002a) and arterial blood gas analysis will need to be done frequently during the first four hours to monitor response. Ventilator pressures and oxygen concentration may require adjusting according to the

Table 8.5. Contraindications to noninvasive ventilation

Coma or confusion
Inability to maintain own airway
Copious amount of respiratory secretions
Nausea or vomiting
Radiological evidence of consolidation
Facial abnormalities (interfere with mask fitting)
Severe COPD unresponsive to relevant therapy
Poor quality of life (housebound)
Malignancy

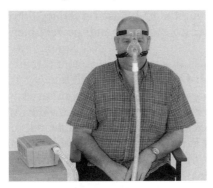

Figure 8.5. Patient using NIV via a nasal mask

blood gas results. Usually the patient's blood gases and condition will show signs of improvement within the first few hours of starting the treatment and may need to continue for at least 24 hours. Normal observations including respiratory rate, pulse and blood pressure will require monitoring. Frequent mouth care or heated humidification may be needed, as the patient may be dry due to the treatment and oxygen administered. If the patient is stable enough, after a few hours the patient should be given a break to drink and eat and take any prescribed medication. The patient will also require basic nursing care and management of an acute patient confined to bed. When the patient is clinically stable and blood gas analysis is more normal the patient can be weaned from the ventilator with the support of supplementary oxygen therapy.

The NICE guidelines (National Collaborating Centre for Chronic Conditions, 2004) also recommend the use of NIV as a treatment for chronic hypercapnic ventilatory failure in selected patients. The evidence suggests that some patients might benefit from such treatment in the long term, combined with LTOT by alleviating fatigued respiratory muscles and improving inspiratory muscle function (Ambrosino *et al.*, 1990). NIV may also reduce hypoventilation associated with desaturation at night (Meecham-Jones *et al.*, 1995), leading to improvements in daytime hypercapnia (Plant and Elliott, 2003). However, the optimal time for starting long-term ventilation is still unclear and the provision of such a service for home NIV is very limited at present. Recommendations for the instigation of NIV in patients with COPD by Meecham-Jones *et al.* (1995) suggest that it should be started where there is evidence of nocturnal hypercapnia, which is responsive to such treatment.

Noninvasive ventilation is an effective treatment for the management of patients admitted with acute hypercapnic respiratory failure. It avoids the need to sedate and mechanically ventilate patients and has reduced the demand for intensive care beds. It has also reduced the complications of tracheal intubation, increased mortality and the length of hospital stay.

LUNG SURGICAL INTERVENTIONS

There remain very few treatment options for patients with end-stage COPD, of which their management can place considerable challenges upon most health professionals. Until recent years surgical treatment has previously been limited and is only an option in a minority of patients. Surgical intervention, such as bullectomy, lung volume reduction surgery (LVRS) and lung transplantation, may be an option for patients with severe COPD, particularly with severe emphysema. Prior to referral patients should have received pulmonary rehabilitation and optimal drug treatment and oxygen therapy. In addition patients should be nonsmokers and without alcohol or drug dependence (Hansel and Barnes, 2004). Relatively recently, surgical procedures to remove functionless areas of damaged lung in patients with COPD have proved to be beneficial in carefully selected patients. Lung transplantation has also been relatively successful in patients with COPD, but availability of organs in the UK is rather limited.

Bullectomy

Bullectomy is the surgical excision of single large bulla that leads to collapse of the surrounding lung tissue (National Collaborating Centre for Chronic Conditions, 2004). The large bullae usually occupy at least one-third of a hemithorax and the excision is commonly performed with video-assisted thoracoscopic surgery (VATS). This procedure is particularly successful in younger patients with the presence of normal or near-normal lung parenchyma surrounding the bullae. The two main indications for this procedure are pneumothorax or severe disabling breathlessness. Major cardiorespiratory contraindications are evidence of hypoxia and hypercapnia and decreased diffusion capacity (Hansel and Barnes, 2004). The best results depend on careful patient selection with improved symptomatic relief and health-related quality of life, which is usually noticed soon after surgery. Operative mortality is relatively low and improvement in lung function and symptoms appear to be maintained for about 5 years (National Collaborating Centre for Chronic Conditions, 2004). However, evidence in one study demonstrated that 9 of 12 patients reviewed 5–10 years following surgery all reported a gradual return of breathlessness with a mean fall of FEV_1 of 82 ml/year, but 5 of the 9 still maintained some of their postoperative improvement. Evidence also suggested that, in general, resection of large bullae does not seem to affect the size of any remaining bullae (National Collaborating Centre for Chronic Conditions, 2004).

Lung Volume Reduction Surgery

Lung volume reduction surgery (LVRS) has recently re-emerged as a surgical option for the treatment of severe COPD as a result of emphysema. The procedure was first introduced in the USA in the 1950s where, since then, the surgical procedure has been modified using modern surgical developments (Young, Fry-Smith and Hyde, 1999). Lung volume reduction surgery involves removing distended and functionless areas of the emphysematous lung. Usually 20–30% of lung tissue is resected. This procedure is usually performed following a bilateral lung resection and stapling through a median sternotomy or by VATS (Argenziano *et al.*, 1997). Unilateral LVRS produces a smaller degree of benefits and may be performed if the lung disease is markedly asymmetrical or if pleural disease prevents a bilateral procedure (Wisser *et al.*, 1997).

Lung volume reduction surgery is not an option for all patients with severe emphysema. However, LVRS may offer an alternative to lung transplantation in selected patients or offer an earlier treatment option as a bridge while awaiting a lung transplant. Patient selection is important and is indicated in patients with severe airflow limitation ($FEV_1 < 30\%$), marked hyperinflation and severe disability despite optimal drug therapy (Halpin, 2003). Patients who have hetergeneous disease on CT are more suitable for LVRS. Contraindications include patients with hypercapnia (>6 kPa) and hypoxia, pulmonary hypertension, gas transfer <30% of predicted value and $FEV_1 < 0.5$ L due to high operative mortality in such patients with severe diseases. Other significant diseases, particularly ischaemic heart disease, also increases risk factors (Hansel and Barnes, 2004).

Assessment for LVRS includes full lung function testing before and after attending a pulmonary rehabilitation programme. Imaging, particularly high-resolution CT scanning, can identify the severity and distribution of emphysema as well as other lung disease. ECG, echocardiography and radionuclide scanning may show the presence and extent of coexistent cardiac disease. Young patients should also be screened for alpha-1 antitrypsin deficiency.

Following lung volume reduction surgery improved efficiency of diaphragmatic and other respiratory muscles, together with increased elastic recoil, have been demonstrated (Sciurba *et al.*, 1996; Criner *et al.*, 1998). As a result of this FEV_1 improves, as well as walking distance and quality of life (National Collaborating Centre for Chronic Conditions, 2004). Longer-term follow-up shows that the peak effect seems to occur at 6–8 months following surgery, after which a slow decline developed. However, after 2 years, most patients will still have better lung function than they had before surgery (Bellamy and Booker, 2003). Overall, LVRS does not appear to have any effect on long-term survival (National Collaborating Centre for Chronic Conditions, 2004).

Lung Transplant

Lung transplantation is an option that may be considered for patients with end-stage COPD and who show a progressive deterioration in quality of life and exercise tolerance (Corris, 1999). Prior to referral, patients should be receiving maximum drug therapy, oxygen therapy if appropriate and have completed a pulmonary rehabilitation programme. Patients with COPD are considered to be potential candidates for a transplant if they meet the following criteria (National Collaborating Centre for Chronic Conditions, 2004):

- $FEV_1 < 25\%$ of predicted (without reversibility).
- And/or $PaCO_2 < 7.3\,kPa$ and/or pulmonary artery pressure with progressive cor pulmonale.
- Preference should be given to patients with elevated $PaCO_2$ with progressive deterioration who require long-term oxygen therapy, as they have the poorest prognosis.

More recently, single lung transplants has become the favoured technique in view of the difficulty in obtaining donor organs; the procedure is technically straightforward. Single lung transplants are usually offered to patients aged less than 65 years and a bilateral lung transplant to patients of less than 60 years as older patents have significantly worse survival rates following transplantation. Generally, patients with deteriorating lung function ($FEV_1 < 25\%$), respiratory failure ($PaCO_2 > 7.3\,kPa$), severe disability and a life expectancy of less than 18 months or onset of cor pulmonale with right ventricular failure would be considered. Contraindications include symptomatic osteoporosis, high or low body mass index, active malignancy, poor renal and hepatic function and previous thoracic surgery due to the risk of haemorrhage (American Thoracic Society, 1998). Use of low-dose prednisolone appears controversial as a contraindication (American Thoracic Society, 1998; Hansel and Barnes, 2004).

The main immediate postoperative complications of lung transplantation are sepsis or diffuse alveolar damage resulting in early mortality. Lung rejection and opportunistic lung infection due to immunosuppressant therapy may also occur. A late and serious complication is the development of obliterative bronchiolitis, which occurs in 30% of patients surviving 5 years (Bellamy and Booker, 2003).

Postoperatively, the functional results of a single lung transplant are acceptable, with most patients achieving an FEV_1 of 50% predicted (Corris, 1999). Bilateral lung transplantation results in greater improvements in FEV_1, but improvements in exercise capacity are not always significantly greater (Trulock, 1998). Regarding prognosis, overall transplants do not appear to improve long-term survival. At one year mortality is around 20% and at five years survival of 50–60% following lung transplantation is significantly lower than other solid organ transplants (Corris, 1999).

The decision of whether to offer lung transplantation to a patient with emphysema is a complex issue and must take into account not only the duration of expected survival but also quality-of-life issues. Patients must also have a strong and positive attitude with a supportive family.

Chapter 9

COPD and Its Effects on Activities of Living

DIFFICULTIES WITH DAILY LIVING

The impact of COPD on an individual patient's daily life, health and well-being can have a devastating effect. As a result patients may experience profound psychological, physical and emotional difficulties. It is important to recognise that once COPD is established, it is both progressive and irreversible, with no curative treatment available. Therefore, the main aim of managing and caring for patients with COPD is to try to improve and preserve their health status and quality of life as far as possible.

During each patient's initial assessment, health professionals will have established which of the symptoms causes patients the most distress and disability, and as a result how it affects their quality of life. As already identified, patients living with COPD report breathlessness as the most severe and distressing symptom. Breathlessness is a subjective experience and appears to have no correlation with an individual patient's lung function. A patient may have an FEV_1 over 1 litre and be unable to perform activities of which a patient with an FEV_1 of less than 500 ml can manage. The potential impact of COPD on individual patients' daily lives can affect them from a physical, psychological and social perspective to varying degrees. As the disease progresses, this consequently causes significant disability, which may profoundly restrict their lives, with loss of independence and social isolation. Patients will vary in how they view and cope with their condition from day to day. Transcripts from two patients demonstrate what life is like for them living with COPD (Tables 9.1 and 9.2).

Table 9.1. Summary of a transcript from a female patient aged 59 living with severe COPD

Life is generally a struggle. At first when I was diagnosed, I did not even know what emphysema was. I'd suffered from bronchitis and asthma for years and have always had phlegm and a slight degree of shortness of breath. I was prescribed inhalers and just accepted my symptoms as the norm. I was able to bring up my family and work as a health care assistant in a nursing home. One day the breathlessness just hit me and I found I could not do the things I was able to do before. I found this very frustrating and depressing and I now wish I had never smoked. At times I want to end it all and have often thought 'what is it all for?'.

The breathlessness is the worst symptom, which causes panic attacks. They really are very frightening experiences. I have learnt to adapt my daily activities and pace myself on my bad days, which are often, usually 3–4 days a week. I have learnt to accept (although it's very hard) that I just can't do things like I used to. On my bad days I use baby wipes to clean myself and don't get dressed as it just takes too much out of me. Even doing this can take me up to half an hour to complete. I feel so embarrassed to admit this. On these days even to make a cup of tea is a struggle. The weather affects my breathing, especially the cold and the wet. Perfumes, air fresheners and flowers also affect me.

I try to do things and be independent around the house. To dust the lounge will take me all morning and I can only manage to Hoover the lounge in stages with rest in between. My family understands, although they were not aware how bad I was for some time, as I would cover my symptoms up or make excuses. I found I am unable to plan things and I really miss doing things with the grandchildren. I usually plan things around my nebuliser times. The installation of my intercom has given me peace of mind. If I am poorly with my breathing, especially at night, at least I can let people in. Before I was really afraid of not being able to let the paramedics into the house because I could not get to open the door.

I feel my quality of life is non-existent and depressing. I'm annoyed about my illness and wish I had never smoked. I feel I'm a prisoner of my illness and find it hard accepting I can't do the things I want. I really miss going into town, which is something I used to do daily. Now I have to rely on my daughter to take me in the car and push me around the supermarket. Everything is just one big struggle, but at least the nebuliser treatment helps my breathing a little.

ASSESSING QUALITY-OF-LIFE ISSUES

The term 'quality of life' can mean different things to different people. Oleson (1990) suggests that it is a subjective perception of satisfaction or happiness with life, which is important to an individual. Alternatively, Bergner (1988) states that it relates to the measurement of physical and emotional function as opposed to physiological function.

To obtain an objective measurement of an individual patient's quality of life, there are various questionnaires available, which address the emotional

Table 9.2. Summary of a transcript from a male patient aged 46 living with severe COPD

Every day is different, but on the whole it is a struggle. Most days are bad, which can be a living nightmare lasting 24–48 hours. Days like this I am unable to do anything except sit in my chair. Even walking a few steps to the toilet makes me breathless. On days like this I restrict my fluids so I don't have to get up so often.

Washing and dressing can be a struggle, but I always make the effort to dress, even on a bad day. It takes me about 45 minutes, resting in between and using my blue inhaler. I have a shower three times a week, but need help from my wife to help with drying, especially my feet.

On my bad days eating can be a problem. Sometimes I'll go several days without eating a meal. I just have soup because trying to eat and breathe is so difficult and tiring.

Before the stair lift was in place I lived downstairs because using the stairs required tremendous effort. When I did get upstairs I was totally wiped out and breathless and unable to do anything. I therefore used to sleep downstairs in the armchair and used the downstairs toilet.

Night times can be really bad. I usually only sleep for an hour or so each night. This has been a long-standing problem. My cough seems to trouble me more than others some nights trying to bring up the phlegm. Sometimes I need to use my inhalers and nebuliser to ease my breathlessness.

I get very annoyed and frustrated with myself because I can't do the things I want to, or go out when I want. I can't plan anything because I don't know how I will be that day. When I am well enough to drive I take my wife shopping. I try and walk round using the supermarket trolley for support, but have to stop frequently to get my breath. Some people stop and stare and think I am some dirty old man, which upsets me.

There are days when I get very low and wonder if there is any point going on. But then I think of my wife and family and that keeps me going. At times I feel embarrassed and frustrated and feel I have lost all my self-dignity. I worry about my wife having to watch me trying to catch my breath, especially on my bad days and am afraid of being a burden to her. I try to hide how I am feeling so she does not worry. You learn different tricks to cover up. I have a very good family and they visit regularly, but I do get upset that I can't play with the grandchildren when they visit, because I get so exhausted. Overall, I try to keep positive and try to cope with my condition. I take the good with the bad. I feel I have a fairly good quality of life, although I would like it to be better, but I have learnt to take things as they come.

and psychological effects of COPD as well as the physical aspects. Validated questionnaires such as the St George's Respiratory Disease Questionnaire (SGRQ) (Jones *et al.*, 1992) and the Chronic Respiratory Questionnaire (CRQ) (Guyatt *et al.*, 1987) are specifically designed for patients with COPD, which quantify the symptoms and the impact of the disease on daily living. Both are quite lengthy and complex, making them unsuitable for daily practice, although these are useful in pulmonary rehabilitation programmes and research studies. The St George's Respiratory Disease Questionnaire has a shortened version, the AQ20 (Barley, Quirk and Jones, 1998), a 20 item 'self-fill' questionnaire, which requires three possible answers, 'yes', 'no' and 'not applicable', that measure health status rather than psychological impact and only takes 2–3 minutes to complete. A further useful questionnaire is the COPD Control Questionnaire (CCQ) (Van Der Molen *et al.*, 2003), which is a short health status questionnaire consisting of 10 questions relating to the patient's symptoms, functional state and mental state, during the past 24 hours or the previous week. This questionnaire enables the health professional and the patient to assess the severity of symptoms and the limitations caused by the disease. It is also a useful tool in measuring and evaluating the effect of treatment on symptoms. Alternatively, the Lung Information Needs Questionnaire (LINQ) (Jones *et al.*, 2004) is a useful tool to assess patients' individual needs for education and to measure the impact of educational initiatives such as pulmonary rehabilitation. The questionnaire consists of 23 questions and takes the patient about 6 minutes to complete. It covers six specific domains: disease knowledge, medicines, self-management, smoking, exercise and diet. The health professional is able to assess the patient's information requirements to enable the patients to manage their own disease effectively.

There are also a number of validated generic psychological assessment scales, not disease-specific, including the Hospital Anxiety and Depression Scale (Snaith and Zigmond, 1994). The Beck Anxiety Inventory (Beck, 1980) and the Beck Depression Inventory (Beck, Steer and Brown, 1986) each consist of 21 items used to assess anxiety and depressive states in patients.

In daily practice, an informal assessment of the patient's quality of life and how COPD infringes on his or her quality of life can be obtained by asking specific questions relating to aspects of the patient's daily life that cause the most distress or difficulties. Questions related to tiredness, fatigue and emotional state, such as anxiety or panic attacks and how the patient deals with symptoms, may be useful. Questions to ask patients may include, for example:

- Do they feel concerned/frightened/anxious/upset regarding their breathlessness?
- Does feeling out of breath make them feel fed up or depressed?
- Do they feel tired?
- Does their breathlessness affect their daily lives and social activities? If so ask what activities are affected.

The answers patients give will provide important information as to the impact of their breathlessness on their psychological wellbeing and daily lives to enable health professionals to help identify individual coping strategies.

COPING STRATEGIES

The main objective in helping patients to live and cope with COPD is to maximise the ability of each patient to live a normal life within the limitations of their disease. For health professionals this entails educating patients to adapt and to enable them to learn to live with their disease. This means encouraging a change of lifestyle, and includes an analysis of how they perform activities and also learning new coping strategies. Patients need to understand that although this condition is not curable, by learning to manage their symptoms they can still enjoy a reasonable quality of life. Understanding why and how their COPD is affecting their lungs and body will enable patients to cope better. For example, understanding that being breathless is not dangerous or harmful will hopefully encourage patients to keep active. Developing such strategies will enable patients to maintain control and autonomy over their condition, rather than allowing the disease to dominate their lives. If patients allow a chronic illness such as COPD to rule their lives and prevent them from going out, it will eventually lead to social isolation, loss of independence and reliance on others. As a result loneliness, depression and anxiety occur.

COGNITIVE BEHAVIOURAL THERAPY

There is growing evidence to suggest that cognitive behavioural therapy (CBT) may be of benefit to patients with chronic lung disease (Lisansky and Clough 1996; Kunik *et al.*, 2001), particularly in patients who experience anxiety or panic attacks when breathless. Cognitive behavioural therapy combines two effective kinds of psychotherapy, cognitive therapy and behavioural therapy, which are based upon the patient's thoughts and reactions that may provoke anxiety or panic attacks. The aim of the cognitive behavioural therapist is to work in partnership with the patient in order to help identify and understand unhelpful patterns of behaviour and thinking that are maintained by the patient's assumptions and beliefs (Heslop and Rao, 2003). The goal of cognitive behavioural therapy is to try and find solutions, by changing the patient's negative thoughts and behaviours into positive thoughts, which will enable the patient to cope more effectively and help to alleviate the response of fear and anxiety when breathless.

ADAPTING DAILY ACTIVITIES OF LIVING

To help identify and discuss further coping strategies that patients can adapt within their daily activities, the Roper, Logan and Tierney model of care (Holland *et al.*, 2003) will be used to cover the various activities of daily living. This model of care provides a useful framework to assess individual patient's physical abilities and needs, to enable the patient to overcome any difficulties and to promote independence. To provide a holistic perspective of care, it is important to add that the health professional may need the support and advice of the multidisciplinary team within the community.

The various activities of living are discussed in turn along with strategies for patients to adopt, to enable them to cope with these daily activities of living. It is hoped that health professionals will be able to discuss such coping strategies with patients when assessing a patient's individual daily needs. It is important for patients with COPD to remember that the key to adapting and coping with daily activities is conservation of energy.

1. Maintaining a Safe Environment

Maintaining a safe environment is essential for an individual's health and wellbeing. For patients with COPD, as their disease progresses their general health may start to deteriorate, affecting their physical, psychological, social, environmental and economic needs. As a result, dependency upon family and friends to provide support in the home may increase. There may be concerns regarding the patient's ability to carry out daily activities safely without risk of falls or accidents, which as a result may have detrimental effects upon the health and quality of life of the patient. Referral to the following agencies or members of the multidisciplinary team should be made, for further assessment regarding installation of aids to assist with daily activities of living that may enable the patient to continue to live within their own home safely may be appropriate:

- Physiotherapist: for assessment regarding mobility aids
- Occupational therapist: for assessment regarding aids, equipment and assistance around the home to help with all activities of living such as washing and dressing, cooking, bed aids, toilet aids, etc.
- Social services: for assessment of help within the home, meals on wheels, grants for alterations in the home such as stair lifts, walk-in showers or outside ramps/lifts to assist with access; benefit entitlement assessment
- Age concern: for assessment of help within the home such as cleaning and shopping

Practical advice to patients relating to keeping things tidy and close to hand to make life easier as well as to conserve energy may be useful. The use of a

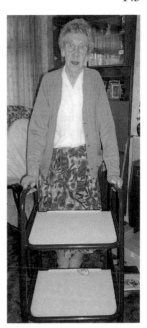

Figure 9.1. Patient using a lightweight trolley

lightweight tray trolley (Figure 9.1) to help transfer items from one place to another may be beneficial, as well as an aid for walking, to avoid accidents and falls.

2. Communication

Communication is an important part of our daily lives. It is essential to remember that communication involves all our vital senses, including our sight and hearing, as well as our mind and memory. As a majority of patients with COPD will be elderly, these vital senses may be affected with the ageing process. It is therefore important to establish the best means of communication for each patient so that they can understand what is being said or communicated to them.

Some patients, particularly with severe COPD, may present with breathlessness at rest, which can affect their ability to communicate effectively and cause them to become tired very quickly. It is useful to encourage breathless patients to talk in short sentences and to pause after each sentence, rather than talking quickly and for long periods before taking a breath. Some patients may be affected if they laugh excessively, causing a breathless attack. Other patients may find talking on the telephone difficult due to their breathlessness, particularly if they rush to answer the phone, which may take them a few minutes to catch their breath. Patients should inform their friends and relatives that they may need time to answer the phone and ensure they sit down while talking. A suggestion of a cordless telephone or a phone placed by their chair to avoid rushing may also help.

3. Breathing

Breathlessness is the worst symptom most patients with COPD experience. They find it distressing and an unpleasant sensation (Davis, 1997). As a result, some patients may enter a cycle of increasing panic and breathlessness, which in turn creates further anxiety. During these severe panic attacks some patients experience the feeling that they are about to die (Davis, 1997). Patients need to be advised of the various measures that they can adopt which will allow them to regain control. These include:

• Providing reassurance and advising the patient to try and stay calm
• Telling them to relax their shoulders, back, neck and arms
• Concentrating on breathing out slowly
• Applying a fan or opening a window to help provide a breeze of air

Other measures for patients to initiate to help control and reduce the degree of breathlessness that they may experience involve adopting energy conservation techniques and learning the art of relaxation.

ENERGY CONSERVATION TECHNIQUES

To reduce aspects of breathlessness, fatigue, anxiety and panic, patients need to be advised on how to conserve their energy to achieve a balance between activities and rest. If patients follow the general principles of energy conservation they will be able to complete tasks without becoming exhausted and gasping for breath within the limitations imposed by their disease. The general principles are as follows.

Pacing activities

Advise patients not to rush activities as this only increases their shortness of breath. The secret is to do things at a slow and steady pace and rest in between tasks, particularly after meals. The use of breathing control during activities will help to reduce the shortness of breath and tiredness. Exhaling during the strenuous part of any activity and the use of pursed-lip and diaphragmatic breathing will reduce the work of breathing.

Planning activities

Advise patients to plan their daily and weekly activities. Where possible patients should do their most strenuous activities when they have the most energy or when they feel their breathing is best during the day. It is advisable to alternate difficult or strenuous activities with easier tasks. It will also help to conserve energy if patients plan and organise the space around them so that things are within easy reach. It is best if things are placed in drawers or shelves that are between the waist and shoulder level to avoid stooping or stretching for items.

General posture

Advise patients where possible to sit down to perform activities in order to consume less energy. Avoid bending down, stretching or lifting, as these positions will increase breathlessness – push, pull or slide instead. If patients need to lift or carry, they should be advised to use their legs and use both hands and carry items close to their body to reduce strain. Maintaining a good position when sitting in a chair or bed uses less effort. Work surfaces should be at the correct height to enable patients to maintain a good posture and to eliminate strain.

Proficiency

Advise patients that organising tasks and daily activities will make life easier and requires less energy. Adapting tasks and using aids or equipment to help will also be beneficial. Overall, patients should be advised to avoid any unnecessary activity.

RELAXATION

Relaxation is an important aspect of learning to cope with living with COPD and with the related symptoms of breathlessness and fatigue. Most patients with COPD are likely to suffer from muscle tension, particularly in their neck and shoulders, due to the way they hold their position and posture to breathe. If patients are stressed, anxious and tense then symptoms of breathlessness and fatigue will be exacerbated as consumption of oxygen is increased. However, it is futile to tell patients they need to relax when they are struggling to catch their breath. Patients need to pre-learn the art of how to relax and how to gain control over the body's response to dealing with stress, anxiety and breathlessness. It is important to explain to patients that they need to learn to control their breathlessness rather than allowing the breathlessness to control them. Relaxation takes time and regular practice to master. However, if patients persevere and remain focused they will feel empowered, as well as feeling much better in themselves and will notice an improvement in their overall symptoms and coping abilities.

Relaxation is a personal activity. Patients need to identify a relaxation technique that they feel comfortable with and that works for them. Such techniques include breathing control, visualisation, music, yoga, meditation, massage and aromatherapy oils.

4. Mobility

Breathlessness and fatigue are the main symptoms that patients experience during exertion, and as a result reduces their mobility. Patients may find when walking that by practising abdominal breathing, they will be less breathless. When walking up stairs, patients will find it easier if they match their breathing with their walking pace by breathing in on one step and out on the next two steps and so on.

Patients with breathlessness will find mobility much easier if they use aids that they can lean on, such as frames or walking sticks. However, patients with severe COPD may require the installation of a stair lift (Figure 9.2) to enable them to manage the stairs or a mobility scooter (Figure 9.3) to help with going out or getting to the shops.

BENDING

Bending over from the waist should be avoided as this makes breathing difficult and can cause breathlessness. To overcome this problem patients should be advised to adopt a crouching position, bending from the knees. If various activities require the patient to work at a low level, such as emptying the

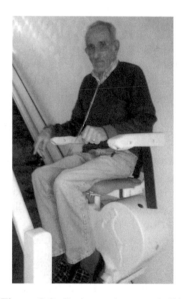

Figure 9.2. Patient using a stair lift

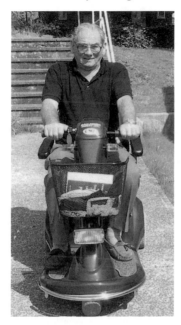

Figure 9.3. Patient using a mobility scooter

washing machine or getting something from a cupboard, then suggest a low stool to sit on to complete the task to avoid bending.

LIFTING HEAVY ITEMS

Carrying heavy items in, for example, shopping bags will restrict the patients' breathing and make breathlessness worse. Therefore, advise patients to distribute the weight and carry items close to their chest or use a rucksack or shopping trolley on wheels.

5. Personal Cleansing and Dressing

Many patients find showering, bathing and dressing particularly tiring. Some patients may even feel panicky and claustrophobic during this activity, increasing their breathlessness. The following suggestions may help to reduce the degree of breathlessness patients may experience and make this activity less strenuous and tiring.

HYGIENE NEEDS

- Advise patients to sit down to wash, shave and brush their teeth. It is best if patients avoid bending down.

- When having a bath or shower, avoid the water being too hot and making the room too steamy. Maybe keep a small window open or the bathroom door open if possible, if not too draughty.
- The use of a nonslip mat in the bath may help. The use of a long-handled back brush to scrub their back as well as their feet makes things easier and less strenuous.
- Sit down while showering, especially if the patient is prone to getting very tired. Position the water spray so that it does not spray directly on to the face to reduce the feeling of breathlessness.
- Advise patients to use an absorbent towelling robe to wrap around them to dry.
- The fitting of grab rails by the bath or shower can be of great help.
- The use of an electric toothbrush is less strenuous.
- Shaving using an electric razor is easier and requires less energy. Avoid shaving creams/foams and after-shave lotions that contain perfume as they may cause a breathless attack.
- If the toilet seat is too low or they find it a struggle, a raised toilet seat or a small grab-rail on the wall will make things much easier for the patient and requires less energy.

DRESSING

- Advise patients to sit down during this activity and to take their time.
- Loose clothing items can be easier to put on and also less restricting on their breathing, particularly around the waist and chest. Avoid the use of tight garments such as bras, girdles and belts. Camisoles may be a better option for women and more comfortable.
- Again advise patients to avoid bending forward. The use of a long-handled shoehorn may be beneficial or slip-on shoes.
- Women may be more comfortable wearing trousers than struggling with nylon tights.
- For both men and women cardigans are easier and less awkward to put on and take off, as stretching and raising their arms above their heads to put a jumper on can be tiring and strenuous. Some women may even prefer a large shawl around their shoulders.

Support may be required from an occupational therapist to assess the patient regarding these activities and the use of various bath aids.

6. Eating and Drinking

Patients with COPD use up more energy to breathe than individuals without this chronic respiratory disease. Therefore they need to replace the calories they burn up by eating a healthy diet. Patients should be advised to eat little and often to avoid getting breathless or bloated after a large meal. Some patients with COPD may even find that trying to eat and breathe is very uncomfortable and exhausting, and are unable to take in adequate nutrition or calories as a result. Other patients may find that increased sputum production, particularly during an exacerbation, affects their sense of taste and appetite.

The following suggestions may help patients with their diet:

- Eat little and often. Use a small main plate to serve meals, as a large portion will be off-putting for patients. If underweight advise three small meals and three snacks, to obtain additional calories to prevent feeling too full and becoming too tired. If overweight, it is important to eat only three small balanced meals a day and not to snack in between.
- Eat foods that require little chewing and are easy to swallow, such as cottage pie, fish pie, omelette, scrambled egg. Foods high in protein are important to help build and repair muscle and tissue.
- Eat a balanced diet with plenty of fresh fruit and vegetables, as these are rich in antioxidants and valuable vitamins and are thought to help protect the lungs.
- Fish should be included in the diet at least twice a week, in particular oily fish, which is high in omega 3 fish oils, as this is thought to protect the lungs due to antioxidants.
- Encourage patients to drink water rather than just cups of coffee and tea, which have a diuretic effect. An adequate water intake of 6–8 glasses per day will also help keep lung secretions thin. This is particularly important if patients are using long-term oxygen therapy. Patients may find it useful to make up small bottles of drink daily and keep them readily available in the fridge or beside them.
- Avoid eating gas-forming foods and carbonated drinks that are likely to cause abdominal distension or a bloated feeling, which may increase breathlessness after a meal. These foods include cabbage, broccoli, cauliflower, beans, asparagus and raw apples.
- Patients who produce a lot of secretions may find that dairy products such as milk, cheese and butter increase this, making expectorating difficult. However, an adequate intake of calcium is required to help towards prevention of osteoporosis.
- Where possible advise patients to sit up to the table to eat their meals. This ensures they are well sat up and not hunched when eating, which will increase their breathlessness.
- If patients become too breathless when eating, they may find it beneficial to apply some oxygen via nasal cannula.
- Avoid lying down at least two hours after eating a meal to avoid the risk of heartburn and acid reflux.

PREPARING AND COOKING MEALS

- Advise patients to prepare easy meals and where possible to avoid pre-packed meals, which have very little nutritional value and are high in salt and additives. Preparing a week's menus may make things easier.
- It may help if patients prepare for a couple of meals and freeze one for another time. This saves time and energy and will only require heating up once defrosted.
- The use of a slow cooker or a pressure cooker can be time saving and easy to use.
- Use lightweight cooking pans and utensils.
- Sit and prepare vegetables, etc.; the use of a perch stool is useful (Figure 9.4).
- When cooking advise patients to have all ingredients laid out to conserve their energy.
- To prevent the kitchen becoming too warm, good ventilation and the use of an extraction fan or portable fan will help.
- If patients find it difficult to prepare meals there are various companies that deliver frozen ready-cooked meals for a week, which just require re-heating.

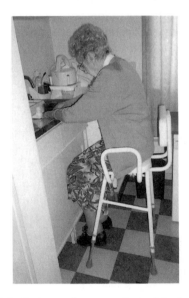

Figure 9.4. Patient using a perch stool in the kitchen

7. Elimination

Getting rid of waste products from our bodies is an essential process to maintain a healthy and balanced metabolism. Problems associated with elimination may impact and compromise many other daily activities of living such as mobilising, eating and drinking, working and playing, expressing sexuality, personal cleansing and dressing, and maintaining a safe environment (Roper, Logan and Tierney, 2000).

MICTURITION

Many patients with COPD may be prescribed diuretics, which cause frequent trips to the toilet. This can be very tiring for the patient, especially if they are breathless on minimal exertion. It may be useful to advise patients to stay in their bedroom near the toilet until the effects of the medication have worn off to save exhausting themselves or to use a commode. Patients should be advised not to omit their diuretics. Older men may suffer from passing frequent small amounts of urine or dribbling or outflow obstruction. One of the commonest causes of urinary retention is seen in males who suffer from benign prostatic disease.

For many women with COPD stress incontinence can be an embarrassing problem, particularly when coughing. Patients may reduce their fluid intake to avoid this problem, which is not advisable and could lead to dehydration, especially in warm weather. Pads can be purchased from the chemist, but if large amounts of urine are void then referral to the district nurse or incontinence service for advice and further assessment should be made.

BOWELS

To avoid constipation patients should be advised to eat a balanced diet, including fruit and vegetables as well as plenty of fluids. Additional fibre may be advisable in the form of bran in cereals or wholemeal bread. Exercise is also essential. Reasons for constipation should be assessed with the patient. Medication may need to be reviewed, as constipation is a common side effect, especially with analgesics such as codeine or opiates.

8. Controlling Body Temperature

Extreme cold or heat is likely to affect patients with COPD regarding their breathlessness. Patients should be advised to take simple measures that can help ensure they remain stable and comfortable.

COLD WEATHER

Patients in cold weather should be advised to only go out if they really have to as bronchospasm is likely to occur when cold air is inhaled, causing breathlessness and wheeze. Cold weather is also associated with viral infections, either by reactivation of latent viruses or due to increased contact with other people with infections. In the winter patients should be advised to do the following:

- If patients have to go out they should ensure they wear several thin layers under their coat and wear gloves, scarf and hat. This is important, as a lot of body heat is lost through the head. Warm shoes or boots with good grips should also be worn.
- When indoors several layers of thin clothing made from wool, polyester or fleecy synthetic fibres are usually warmer. Thermal underwear with warm, thick tights or long socks will also help to keep patients warm. As patients with severe COPD are less likely to be very active, a shawl around their shoulders or a blanket over the knees will provide a lot of warmth.
- The living room and bedroom temperature should be maintained at about 21 °C. Double glazing, insulation and draughtproofing will help keep bills down. Patients may be entitled to a grant to complete these energy-efficient schemes.

WARM WEATHER

Patients with COPD are also likely to suffer in the summer due to the heat and may experience an increase in breathlessness as well as symptoms of hayfever if high pollen counts affect them. In the summer patients should be advised to do the following:

- Stay indoors in extreme heat and keep windows closed if affected by hayfever.
- Keep curtains closed to keep the room cool.
- Wear lightweight clothing.
- An electric fan may help patients to keep cool and avoid breathless attacks.
- Patients should be advised to drink plenty of water to prevent becoming dehydrated.

9. Sleeping

Sleep is vital for all individuals in order to restore energy and body growth and to wake feeling refreshed. For patients with COPD breathlessness, cough and difficulty in expectorating can affect the quantity and quality of sleep.

The amount of sleep each patient needs may vary for each individual. Older people tend to sleep for shorter periods at night and may tend to wake more frequently during the night for a number of reasons that may not be specifically related to their COPD, such as needing to go to the toilet, pain or discomfort from arthritis.

Hypnotic drugs may be an option that patients may wish to discuss with their GP, but where possible these should only be used for short periods due to the high risk of depressing the respiratory centre and addictive factors. The following suggestions may be helpful in advising patients in obtaining a restful night's sleep:

- To help with symptoms of breathlessness or cough patients should be advised to use their inhaler or nebuliser prior to going to bed.
- Avoid caffeine, nicotine and alcohol in the evening. Take a glass of water to bed to help ease any cough or dryness.
- Having a warm milky drink before going to bed may help.
- Ensure the bedroom is comfortable and at the desirable temperature for sleeping.
- If breathless the patient will need to sit up well supported by pillows in bed.
- The use of a quilt rather than sheets and blankets is desirable.
- A fan may be useful if the patient wakes up breathless during the night.
- Inhaler and medication should be at hand, to avoid the patient panicking during a breathless attack.
- Take some form of analgesia before going to bed if pain is a cause for poor sleep.
- Reading a book or playing some relaxing music may help the patient to sleep.
- In the morning, patients should be advised not to leap out of bed, but to take their time by sitting on the edge of the bed first and using their 'blue' inhaler (Salbutamol).

10. Expressing Sexuality

Roper, Logan and Tierney (1996) view sexuality as more than sex and sexual intercourse, which they consider an important component of adult relationships. Each individual has their own personal view of what it means to them and refers to sexual expression in the form of sexual feelings and beliefs. Being close and feeling loved is an essential activity in any relationship and is no different for a patient with COPD. Heath professionals may feel embarrassed or uncomfortable discussing such issues with patients and may shy away from this topic or they may not consider this aspect of their patients' lives as relevant. However, patients and their partners should be offered the opportunity to discuss their fears and anxieties relating to this subject. Just because a patient has COPD does not mean that this aspect of their lives should just become a memory. Health professionals may need to initiate this topic of conversation during an assessment.

Patients with COPD may experience a wide range of symptoms including breathlessness, cough, sputum production, wheeze, fatigue, anxiety and depression. Each of these may have some degree of impact on the patient's sexual activity from either a physical or psychological perspective (Law, 2001). It is important to emphasise to patients that as long as the breathlessness is not uncomfortable and can be tolerated then it is not harmful. Patients may need to talk to their partner to discuss ways they can adapt and enjoy this activity. The following practical suggestions may be helpful for patients to consider:

- Advise patients to plan this activity when they are at their best if possible.
- Avoid having sex in the morning as this is when most patients are not at their best.
- Avoid having sex after a heavy meal or alcohol.
- Advise patients to use their bronchodilator 15 minutes prior to sexual activity.
- Use oxygen if prescribed during sexual activity.
- Clear bronchial secretions beforehand.
- Keep the room at a comfortable temperature.
- Start slowly and take regular rests.
- Advise patients to chose sex positions that are less energy consuming and that avoid pressure on the chest. Where possible the patient should encourage their partner to assume a more active role so that they do not become too tired or breathless.
- Avoid perfumes, aftershave or aerosols, which may induce bronchospasm.
- Above all, patients should communicate with their partner and remember that the intimacy of kissing and cuddling is as important as sexual intercourse.

For patients that still have unanswered questions or concerns referral to their GP or a sexual therapist for professional counselling may be required.

11. Working and Playing

On average most people spend about two-thirds of their working day engaged in activities that are associated with working and playing. It gives each of us a sense of purpose in life whether it is going to work or staying at home and doing the housework. Playing is considered equally important and focuses upon activities that are conducted during each individual's spare time.

WORK

Patients still in employment when diagnosed with COPD may need support and advice depending on the type of occupation they are employed in. It will very much depend on the severity of the patients' symptoms and the physical energy required to complete their job, as to whether they are able to continue in their present occupations. Patients may be faced with various dilemmas if they have to give up work, with the loss of a daily routine as well as the loss of social interaction with work colleagues. Further repercussions for patients regarding loss of earnings and personal independence will have an impact on their lives. Patients should contact social services for advice regarding benefits they may be entitled to claim should this situation arise. To prevent depression and frustration developing patients should be encouraged to continue, or consider, taking up hobbies to keep them active, preferably with a friend or partner for company.

HOUSEHOLD TASKS

Patients may feel guilty and frustrated about the inability to perform domestic tasks around the house and in the garden. Patients therefore need to learn to adapt and divide tasks into manageable chunks. They need to learn to plan activities and take frequent breaks. It may take them that much longer, but at least they will have achieved their goal. For heavier tasks such as hoovering it is best to invest in a lightweight vacuum cleaner. If patients are unable to perform this task then some paid help or a member of the family can do this instead. Damp dusting is advised rather than the use of spray polishes and a long-handled duster should be used for high areas. Advise patients to reduce clutter and ornaments that only collect dust, which will reduce the amount of cleaning required.

GARDENING

Patients can still pursue their gardening if this is a hobby they enjoy. Reducing the amount of lawn and laying slabs or chipping's will reduce the worry of mowing the lawn and will look tidy. Patients can plant bedding plants in small pots or tubs, which can easily be done while sitting down in order to conserve energy. Raised flowerbeds are also another alternative and the use of long-handled tools will help.

EFFECTS ON SOCIAL ACTIVITIES

Impaired activity levels due to breathlessness associated with COPD can have a significant impact on both the patient and their partner, family and carers. It can reduce their ability to socialise, take holidays and enjoy a normal life.

Patients may find social activities very exhausting and may take several days to recover. Patients should be advised to plan ahead, pace themselves and avoid rushing, which will otherwise result in panic and induce breathlessness. Patients should avoid smoky environments and avoid going out in very cold and wet weather. Patients should also be advised to use their bronchodilator before they go out and to carry their inhaler with them.

Holidays

Holidays can still be planned even though patients have COPD. Patients must be realistic as to where they go and the type of holiday they want. Planning in advance is vital, taking into consideration wheelchair access, how far they can walk, the number of stairs/steps they can manage, access to toilets and what transport they can use. Adequate medication must be taken and provision made for oxygen and nebuliser therapy if required. An emergency supply of antibiotics and steroids is also a good idea, which the patient can start immediately if they present with an exacerbation of their COPD, as well as seeking medical advice.

Effects on Relationships

Carers perform a vital role in caring for patients with this chronic disease, which can be stressful and demanding. The stress, physical and emotional effects of COPD are likely to have an impact on family relationships. Roles within the family unit may reverse as a result. It is inevitable therefore that at some stage partners and carers will feel anxious, frustrated or even resentful towards the patient, especially if the patient is totally dependent on them. A transcript from a carer demonstrates this (Table 9.3). Where possible, it is important to tell the family and carers that the patient should be encouraged to remain as independent for as long as possible and to enjoy things together (Figure 9.5).

Being a carer can be emotionally and physically taxing. Day-to-day help can be obtained from social services or private agencies. Regular breaks should be encouraged for full-time carers to enable them to have some respite and to recharge their 'batteries'. This may be in the form of a few hours a week to go into town or to visit a friend for coffee. Respite may also be offered to patients while carers go away on holiday. Family and friends are important for carers in providing them with the additional emotional support they may require.

Support Groups

The British Lung Foundation provides information and support to patients and carers with lung disease. It offers an extensive range of information booklets, leaflets and fact sheets.

Table 9.3. Summary of a transcript from a female carer looking after her husband with severe COPD

I have been a full-time carer for the last 5 years. I had to give up my part-time job, which I loved, to look after my husband, John. At the time I did feel rather resentful and I still miss the company. My husband is now housebound and has had to sell his car, as he can no longer drive. This makes shopping quite difficult, especially to do a big shop, as I suffer from arthritis myself and have back problems. I do use the internet to help with my shopping but its not the same as visiting the shops and picking out your own fresh produce. My neighbour will help by getting the odd item for me.

My day can start as early as 4 am some days if my husband wakes up early and is breathless. I have to get up to give him his nebuliser and to make sure he is ok. The day is taken up with seeing to my husband and helping him with various tasks he can't do. Things have to be done in John's own time, which can sometimes take ages to do simple little things. This can be frustrating at times when I have things I need to get done. To plan for a bath can take an hour or so to initiate and then a further hour to actually have a bath and complete the task. Meal times can be a problem and frustrating. I can stand and prepare a meal, something John likes and then most of it goes in the bin because he can't eat it and you feel you are cooking for nothing.

I go out for a couple of hours each week into town on the bus. I make sure John is ok before I go and that he has had all his medication. But I can never totally relax when I am out because I am constantly wondering if he is all right. I also phone him on my mobile to check. I can't really plan anything with a friend in advance because I don't know how John is going to be each day. If he is having a bad day then I can't go out. I go and have my hair done each week, but I leave the house at 7 am after seeing to John and making sure he is ok and am back by 8.30 am. So in total I only have 9 hours out a week, but it is not quality time because half of that is spent on the bus. At times I really feel trapped and frustrated and feel I am clock watching all the time. We have one son but he lives away. I have a couple of really good friends, but I don't like to trouble them. If I need any jobs doing around the house like electrical or plumbing then I have a friend's husband I can call upon; otherwise I have to pay someone to do the job. I try to do most things myself. I do all the jobs in the garden and what decorating I can manage.

We are not able to take holidays together now, as John can't walk very far and we can't go to my son's, as he does not have a stair lift or a downstairs toilet. I go away for a week once a year to Blackpool with my friend, while John goes into respite. He was very apprehensive last year when he went but now he knows the staff he is quite looking forward to it this year. I do get low, at screaming point sometimes. I could do with a second break each year but I don't have anyone else I could go with and I don't want to go away on my own. I would not enjoy that. John does not want to go to a day centre for the day, which would free me up for a day.

If John gets into a panic when he is breathless he is difficult to reassure and wants me to call the ambulance. I feel panicky myself, but have to try and keep calm for John's sake. Life can be difficult but I try to cope the best I can and keep things as normal as possible.

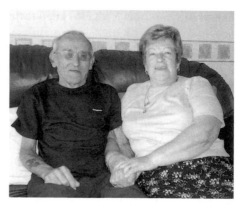

Figure 9.5. Patient and carer

The Breathe Easy Club, which is organised by the British Lung Foundation, provides practical support to patients and carers. Most areas have a local group who meet on a regular basis, and are a valuable social and educational resource. These groups offer the chance to meet and share experiences with other people with lung disease.

12. Dying

Death is a process that inevitably occurs to us all. However, when and how this event occurs is an unknown phenomenon. COPD is an incurable disease with a poor prognosis, which gradually deteriorates over time. Unlike patients with incurable cancer, it is impossible to speculate how long patients are likely to survive with COPD once it reaches the severe stage. Many patients survive several years with extremely poor lung function and disability. Patients with deteriorating COPD often develop various co-morbid conditions and complications associated with this condition and smoking.

It is important to develop a good therapeutic relationship with patients and their families, where an honest and open relationship can be formed. Patients who feel supported and have established trusting partnerships are likely to seek information about their deteriorating condition and what they may expect towards the end of their lives. Patients may experience various emotional responses during the terminal stage of their illnesses, such as denial, anger, anxiety and depression (Twycross, 1999). Health professionals will need to help the patients work through these phases to enable them to accept what is happening and to cope with their feelings.

Effective management of symptoms is vital to keep the patient comfortable and to preserve each individual's dignity and quality of life. Appropriate liaison with the palliative care team may be required to help facilitate this area of care. Involving the patient and their family in the management and care is essential, especially if the patient wants to stay at home.

Chapter 10

Palliative Care in Patients with COPD

WHAT IS PALLIATIVE CARE?

Palliative care is the active, total care of patients and their families whose condition is no longer responsive to curative treatments (World Health Organisation, 2002). Palliative care focuses on symptom control, psychosocial and spiritual care, and development of a personalised management plan to provide the patients with some quality of life (Billings, 2000). It is an area of care that involves the active and coordinated involvement of members of the multidisciplinary team, the patient and family members in all care decisions. However, within COPD, palliative care is an area of care that is sadly neglected and not readily available. Care and management of COPD appears to concentrate mainly on acute exacerbations. However, we know that 32 000 patients die a year from this disease and that over 10% of all acute admissions are related to COPD. A recent audit of 1400 patients admitted to hospital with an exacerbation showed that 14% had died within 3 months (Roberts *et al.*, 2002). The prognosis for many patients with COPD is poor, with a reduced quality of life. Like many nonmalignant conditions, the rate of deterioration is difficult to predict and may extend into decades. The principles of palliative care are therefore an integral component in delivering good clinical care and symptom control. Palliative care should provide holistic care to patients with a noncurable disease, such as COPD, and should include addressing their health and social needs. Many of the symptoms COPD patients experience or suffer are not unlike those with a malignant lung disease. Although symptoms in patients with cancer may be more severe, those patients with a non-malignant condition tend to be more prolonged (O'Brien, Welsh and Dunn, 1998) and chronic. However, the provision of palliative care services to this group of patients is less well developed and appears to be almost exclusively confined to malignant disease (Eve, Smith and Tebbit, 1997). A study conducted by Gore, Brophy and Greenstone (2000) compared the needs of patients with COPD and those with lung cancer. It suggested that patients with end-stage COPD, who had a significantly impaired quality of life and emotional wellbeing, did not receive the holistic care appropriate to their needs compared to those with lung cancer. Patients with COPD received no specialist care compared to 30% of those patients with lung cancer who received help from specialist palliative care services. Interestingly, 90% of the COPD patients in this study suffered from anxiety and depression compared to 52% of patients with lung cancer. Although very few studies have been completed relating to palliative care approaches in COPD, those of us that care for this group of patients would not be surprised by the findings above and are more than aware that the provisions of care could be much better.

WHEN TO IMPLEMENT PALLIATIVE CARE?

Deciding when a patient has reached the stage where palliative care is required is often difficult to determine, as this will vary from patient to patient depending on the severity of their symptoms and the rate of decline. In patients with end-stage COPD it is usually considered to be the point at which long-term containment of the disease is no longer possible (Rose, 1995). It is therefore vital that these patients should have access to the full range of services offered by the multidisciplinary palliative care teams (National Collaborating Centre for Chronic Conditions, 2004), which are likely to vary greatly between geographical areas. Developing such links and integrating these services would certainly enhance the care and management of patients with this disease and enable them to optimise their quality of life as well as enhancing the individual heath professional's own knowledge and skills.

Patient Choice

The care and management of patients with end-stage COPD initially lies with health professionals within primary care. Patients should be kept informed of their condition and prognosis so that their treatment and management can be discussed. Adequate and appropriate palliative care requires a planned and coordinated approach to ensure that it is provided at the right time and in the right place. Patients needing palliative care should be able to choose where they spend their final days. Although most patients may wish to die at home, only a small percentage may achieve this wish. Patients with COPD, unlike those with lung cancer, may go from crisis to crisis, and as a result require an increased number of hospital admissions and are therefore more likely to die in hospital (Edmonds, 2001). Nonetheless, it is important to ensure that the passage through this stage of a patient's illness is as stress free and as comfortable as possible. Forward planning and collaborative team working can avoid unwanted complications or problems arising and enable the patient to have a peaceful death at home surrounded by loved ones. However, the desired place of death may change if symptoms and care or practical support is inadequate. Patients who are frightened, insecure or lack confidence in their support network are more likely to need urgent hospital admission. Equally, if carers are struggling or are either physically or mentally tired, hospital admission may be appropriate, even when death is imminent (O'Neill and Rodway, 1998).

ADVANCE DIRECTIVES

The availability today of advanced medical technology to prolong life is very much evident. However, patients who have severe COPD may want to be given the choice of whether they receive advanced or aggressive treatment should their condition deteriorate suddenly. This, in particular, relates to cardiopulmonary resuscitation and artificial ventilation. Advance directives allow individuals to express their wishes regarding their treatment or future healthcare in the event of them becoming incompetent and unable to give consent. A directive can be made, preferably in writing, to decline a specific treatment or to indicate their wishes of where they are treated either at home or in hospital. Interestingly, a study conducted by Gaber *et al.* (2004) surveyed 100 patients with moderate or severe COPD in the community regarding their views on cardiopulmonary resuscitation and noninvasive ventilation. Forty-eight patients acknowledged they would want both cardiopulmonary resuscitation and noninvasive ventilation. Nineteen patients said 'no' to cardiopulmonary resuscitation but 'yes' to noninvasive ventilation or other intervention if required, and ten patients said 'no' to cardiopulmonary resuscitation but would accept noninvasive ventilation. Twelve patients stated they would not want any kind of intervention and the remaining eleven gave mixed answers.

Patients should be encouraged to discuss such issues if they wish and all the options available to them should be explained, either with their GP or any other health professional involved in their care. Choosing the right time to discuss such matters can, however, be difficult to decide. Nonetheless, patients are becoming more knowledgeable and open in their approach and may initiate this issue independently with health professionals.

Advance directives should be written clearly and signed by the patient and a witness, who should not be a member of the family. A copy should then be filed in the patient's medical notes and with the GP. Any advance directive should be reviewed annually. The common core content of an advance directive should contain the following (Watson *et al.*, 2005):

- Patient's name and address
- Name and address of GP
- A clear statement of the patient's wishes
- Name, address and contact number of the next of kin
- Signatures of the patient and witness and dated

STRATEGIES FOR IMPROVING SYMPTOM CONTROL

The key principles underpinning palliative care comprise focusing on achieving good symptom control and enhancing the patient's quality of life to the end. Such interventions are noncurative treatments, which enable the patient to either control or increase their coping strategies in managing their symptoms better. The most common symptoms associated with end-stage COPD are severe breathlessness, cough and fatigue. These symptoms and their management in palliative care are discussed in turn.

Breathlessness

Breathlessness is a frightening symptom that may be exacerbated with anxiety and panic attacks, particularly in the end stage of COPD. Many patients will therefore avoid activities that may bring on these attacks and as a result become deconditioned and more dependent on carers.

It is important for health professionals to conduct a thorough assessment to exclude any other causes for breathlessness other than severe COPD, such as pleural effusion, pneumothorax, pneumonia, lung cancer, anaemia or heart failure, which may be effectively treated to relieve the breathlessness to some extent. A clinical assessment tool, known as the Breathlessness Assessment Guide, can be used to assess the severity of their breathlessness and the impact this has on their daily lives (Corner and Driscoll, 1999). This will enable a clear picture to be obtained so appropriate practical advice on various coping strategies can be provided.

NONPHARMACOLOGICAL MANAGEMENT

Providing practical advice to patients and carers is important. This should include an explanation of their symptoms to enable patients to feel in control. Advice on the use of a fan to provide a cool stream of air over the patient's face can reduce the sensation of breathlessness and assist in the avoidance of a panic attack. The adoption of a good position, well sat up, supported by pillows will help. Carers should be taught to stay calm, to reassure and talk the patient through any panic attacks. Relaxation techniques and breathing control exercises taught by a physiotherapist may be helpful.

Optimal doses of bronchodilators should be administered. If patients are unable to manage inhalers via a spacer or require larger doses, then a nebuliser should be tried to deliver the medication. Oral corticosteroids may help if the patient is particularly wheezy and, as an added bonus, may also help improve the patient's appetite and wellbeing. Theophyllines may be useful in reducing the sensation of breathlessness in the absence of any bronchodilator effect. However, it is important to bear in mind the potential interactions with certain drugs including cimetidine, ciprofloxacin and erythromycin and the fact that the half-life may be increased in patients with heart failure or hepatic impairment.

Opioids, such as Oramorph®, may be of benefit, particularly if patients are very anxious. Morphine works by reducing the excessive respiratory drive and substantially reduces the ventilatory response to hypoxia and hypercapnia. By slowing the respiratory rate, breathing may be made more efficient, and the sensation of breathlessness reduced (Watson *et al.*, 2005). If patients are unable to swallow, drug treatment can be administered using a subcutaneous infusion via a syringe driver. Patients taking opiates should be given a laxative to overcome the side effects of constipation.

Anxiety and fear often accompany breathlessness. Panic attacks with hyperventilation and the fear of suffocation worsen the sensation of breathlessness. Anxiolytics may help to reduce anxiety. Buspirone, which does not suppress respiration, may be of benefit or low doses of benzodiazepines such as lorazepam or diazepam. Any concern regarding respiratory depression should be weighed against the potential benefit of treatment (Davis, 1997).

Oxygen therapy may help breathlessness in patients, particularly if they are hypoxic at rest or post-exertion. Short-burst therapy may be of benefit to patients with extreme breathlessness and reduced oxygen saturations post-exertion. However, for patients who are not hypoxic there is no evidence to support the use of oxygen in palliative care (Davis, 1997). Many patients become highly dependent on oxygen therapy, which provides more of a psychological placebo, and the cooling effect of the gas from the cylinder. It is therefore important to assess and evaluate the benefits from a subjective and objective perspective for each patient individually.

Cough

A cough is the normal physiological mechanism that naturally protects the airways and lungs by removing mucus or foreign matter. In patients with nonmalignant and malignant lung disease a pathological cough is common. For some patients their cough can be just as distressing and frightening as breathless attacks. Very severe coughing fits may induce syncope or vomiting and some patients may lose control of their bladder or bowels. Constant coughing will cause muscular skeletal strain in the chest wall, exhaustion, lack of sleep and some patients may even suffer fractured ribs.

During assessment it is important to identify whether the patient has a productive, wet or dry cough and if there are any reversible causes that require treatment. If the patient has a productive cough it is useful to identify the colour of their sputum and if they report any signs of haemoptysis.

MANAGEMENT OF A PRODUCTIVE/WET COUGH

Firstly, identify whether the patient has a chest infection and treat appropriately with antibiotics. Nebulised bronchodilators may help reduce bronchospasm. Patients with problems expectorating tenacious sputum may find nebulised sodium chloride 0.9% of benefit by loosening up the secretions. Mucolytics, which aim to reduce the viscosity of mucus such as carbocysteine, are worth trying for a month. Other simple methods to help with expectorating are steam inhalations using menthol crystals or friars balsam. Advise patients not to use a towel as the steam may induce a breathless attack. Patients using continuous oxygen may find this particularly drying if using four or more litres per hour. Humidification may be of benefit.

It is important to ensure that patients continue to take in adequate fluids if possible. A good posture and breathing exercises and huffing will also help with expectorating. Physiotherapy may also benefit if the patient is not too frail. For patients who are in the last few days of life, and too weak to expectorate, it may be more appropriate and more comfortable for the patient to be given hyoscine hydrobromide as a subcutaneous injection or by subcutaneous infusion to help to reduce mucus secretions (Davis, 1997).

MANAGEMENT OF A DRY COUGH

Cough suppressants can be suggested to patients if no other underlying cause can be found. For throat irritation simple linctus (in warm water) may help. Another central cough suppressant is codeine linctus, a mild antitussive that may be used if patients are not already on opioids, which causes less sedation (Watson *et al.*, 2005).

Fatigue

Fatigue is a common and debilitating symptom for all patients suffering from severe COPD. As a result, this can have a profound effect on their quality of life, causing a decreased ability to perform daily activities of living independently. Fatigue is a subjective experience, which can leave the patient extremely tired with an overwhelming desire to rest and sleep (Trendall, 2000). Although a common symptom, there appears to be a lack of literature specifically related to patients with COPD. Much of the literature available is related to patients with cancer, neurological problems, chronic fatigue syndrome, radiotherapy and patients who have undergone surgery (Trendall, 2001). The fatigue many patients experience is obviously linked to the additional effort required for patients to breathe. Patients with end-stage COPD are usually weak and frail with a significant degree of muscle wasting, which is likely to affect the working efficiency of their respiratory muscles. Patients are also likely to use accessory muscles to assist with their breathing, requiring a greater consumption of oxygen.

It is important if patients complain of fatigue as a symptom to identify how it is affecting them and their ability to function both mentally and physically. Initially, look to see if there are other contributing factors other than their COPD that may be attributing to their fatigue. For example, it may be that they are not sleeping well at night, are in pain, feel depressed or may have other medical conditions such as anaemia, infection or an electrolyte imbalance that may need correcting. The patient's medication should also be checked to ensure that this is not a cause, and any nonessential medication should be reviewed.

Nursing interventions to assist patients experiencing fatigue should include energy conservation and pacing of activities as well as breathing control exercises to help alleviate their symptoms. Explaining the effects of why they feel drained or are lacking energy will provide patients with reassurance. The importance of keeping active and being realistic as well as providing coping strategies, as discussed in the previous chapter, will also be of help. Any underlying depression should be treated to enable patients to cope better with their symptoms. Attention to nutritional intake is important. However, at this stage, patients may require additional nutritional supplements in the form of Ensure or Enlive drinks if their appetite is really poor.

CARERS

Many patients, without the support of family and friends, would be unable to remain at home until the end. It can be a distressing and stressful time for carers. They will require detailed information and education regarding the patient's condition and any equipment that is used to keep the patient comfortable, as well as how to care for the patient. They will need to be informed of the patient's likely diagnosis and the course of events leading to their death. Carers who are well informed and prepared are more likely to cope better and will also help to allay any anxieties they may have. Some carers may find it a burden caring for a dying relative and others will find the experience rewarding, especially knowing that they have fulfilled the patient's wish to die at home rather than in hospital. However, during this process it may place a great strain on the carers, both emotionally and physically. Carers should be involved in any decisions regarding the patient's care and management and

Table 10.1. Summary of a transcript from a female carer who looked after her husband during end-stage COPD

Initially my husband was sent home from hospital following a severe exacerbation of COPD and pneumonia where I was informed that he only had six weeks or so to live. However, I looked after my husband at home for over nine months.

During those nine months I had the support of the one-to-one service that sat with my husband while I went into town to do my shopping and the COPD nurse specialist who visited weekly. The advice and support from both services I found invaluable. My husband's GP was also very supportive. I managed all my husband's nursing needs and managed his medication, including the administration of his oxygen, which was delivered via an oxygen concentrator, and his nebulised therapy, which he required four times a day.

Caring for my husband 24 hours a day, seven days a week was very tiring, especially as my husband woke every night at 3 am needing his nebuliser, which I needed to give him. I found it very hard watching my husband fading away before my eyes. A lot of the time I felt afraid, sad, and lonely. When he became extremely breathless he would have panic attacks and at times I would feel so helpless. During the nine months my husband received respite care to enable me to have a break and time to recharge my batteries.

Unfortunately, because of a fall he had, I was unable to keep him at home. He was transferred to a nursing home where he died three days later. I felt very guilty and upset about this but I could not manage him on my own as he was so immobile. However, I know I did my best to look after him and that it was my love for him that gave me the strength to keep going.

---

their opinions listened to. A transcript from a wife who cared for her husband during the end stage of his illness (Table 10.1) illustrates her experiences and feelings.

It is important to provide the patient with as much support as possible and to emphasise to the carers that they are not alone. Providing them with contact numbers and information on services that are available, especially in an emergency, will be helpful. These include services from the district nurses, Macmillan nurses and clinical nurse specialists. The Marie Curie nurses provide night sitting services and respite care may be available at local hospices. A thorough assessment should be done to ensure that all additional aids and appliances required are supplied by the occupational therapist or physiotherapist. Additional financial assistance or home care help should be referred to social services.

The ultimate goal is to ensure that the patient has a peaceful and dignified death in a calm and relaxed atmosphere at home, if this is their wish, surrounded by loved ones. Carers should acknowledge that they helped achieve the patient's wish to die at home, which ought to provide them with much comfort during their bereavement. Carers can feel at a great loss after the event. It is important that a visit is made by a health professional after the funeral to discuss any issues the carer may have and to 'close' the relationship that they may have formed during this time. Counselling may be advised for the carer if particularly distressed or is finding the death difficult to deal with.

COMPLEMENTARY THERAPIES

An interest in complementary therapies has increased over the last few years, not just as an alternative to conventional medicine but also for use in conjunction with orthodox medicine in order to provide a more holistic approach to care. The primary aim of complementary therapies is to provide comfort and a sense of wellbeing by promoting relaxation, reducing stress and anxiety, and may help in relieving pain and other symptoms. The central belief of complementary therapy is the strong belief in the uniqueness of the individual and the body's natural healing powers (Watson *et al.*, 2005) to maintain harmony within the body.

Although it has been suggested that one in five people in the UK use complementary therapies (Whitehead, 2003), very little research has been conducted to produce evidence-based facts that it is effective or has any real value, particularly in COPD. Complementary treatments may be sought for chronic illness, probably as a result of conventional medicine no longer being effective or offering relief. The most widely practised complementary therapies in the UK are osteopathy, chiropractic, homeopathy, acupuncture and herbalism (Lewith, 1998). Herbalism is the most accessible because of the availability of these products in high street chemists, supermarkets and health food shops (Kroll, 2001). However, herbal remedies do need to be used with caution, particularly if taking conventional medication, in order to avoid adverse drug reactions (Lewith, 1998).

Other complementary therapies such as reflexology, Indian head massage and aromatherapy massage are becoming increasingly popular in promoting relaxation and reducing stress and anxiety, and are offered in most hospice settings in the UK (Vickers, 2000). Music therapy and visualisation are beneficial therapies that patients can initiate themselves at home to help relieve stress and anxiety, particularly if associated with panic attacks.

Complementary therapies may certainly have a place for patients with COPD and in palliative care from the perspective of helping induce relaxation and a sense of wellbeing. Relaxation techniques used to manage breathlessness in patients with lung cancer demonstrated a reduction in physical and emotional distress combined with improved coping strategies, despite generally deteriorating (Bredin, 1998). In addition, complementary therapies also provide patients with a greater sense of choice and control than they might achieve with conventional treatment alone (Watson *et al.*, 2005).

Unfortunately, many of these therapies are not available on the NHS. Therefore there is a need for more research to be conducted in this field to provide evidence of the effectiveness in the management of symptoms within respiratory medicine.

Chapter 11

Specialist Support within Primary Care for Patients with COPD

THE ROLE OF THE SPECIALIST NURSE

Until very recently COPD has had a very poor image. In the past patients with this condition were often stereotyped and largely viewed as hopeless cases where little could be done for them. Thankfully, things are changing for patients with COPD. Although we cannot offer a cure, we know that appropriate intervention and treatment can slow the rate of decline and vastly improve a patient's quality of life. The development of the COPD guidelines from NICE (National Collaborating Centre for Chronic Conditions, 2004) and the implementation of the General Medical Services (GMS) Contract have helped to raise the profile of the disease and to set a benchmark of care and management for these patients.

The role of caring for patients with COPD varies up and down the country depending on the resources available. However, most large areas are likely to have in post a COPD nurse specialist or a respiratory nurse specialist with an interest in COPD, to carry out this role in the community. As already identified, many patients with COPD have specific needs, which may be complex, and can benefit significantly from expert intervention to manage their condition.

The prime role of the nurse specialist is initially to stabilise the patient's symptoms and optimise medical treatment, ensuring that he or she is compliant and use the medication correctly. Provision of support, advice and education is extremely important in providing the patient and carers with appropriate information about the patient's condition. Helping patients to understand about their condition, how their medication works and why they develop symptoms is paramount to enable patients to manage their condition effectively.

The specialist nurse has a valuable role to play in listening and talking to patients with regards to how living with COPD impacts on their daily lives and how this affects their quality of life. Assisting the patient to identify various coping strategies to overcome these difficulties is vital in enabling the patient to come to terms with the condition.

The nurse specialist is also responsible for monitoring the patient's respiratory status by conducting a respiratory assessment. This will include recording the patient's pulse and respiratory rate, spirometry, pulse oximetry and dyspnoea score. Advice on health promotion issues such as diet, exercise and smoking cessation should also be included.

Effective patient care, however, requires a collaborative approach with members of the multidisciplinary team within the community, which the specialist nurse may initiate if required. These may include a physiotherapist, occupational therapist, dietician, social worker, behaviour nurse therapist or clinical psychologist.

Although research on the role of the specialist nurse in COPD is scarce (National Collaborating Centre for Chronic Conditions, 2004), there is evidence to suggest that there are benefits within this role. Patients cared for by a specialist nurse within the community are helped by gaining reassurance that they are not alone, which enhances their confidence (Barnett, 2003). Patients report that their symptom control is improved (Barnett, 2003) as well as their quality of life and their independence increases (Niziol, 2004). Carers also appreciate the support and advice (Niziol, 2004). There is evidence that specialist nurses are effective in reducing hospital admissions as patients can be managed effectively at home, thereby reducing pressure on hospital beds and reducing A&E admissions (Barnett, 2003; Niziol, 2004). This results in a reduction of pressure on GP services such as surgery consultation time and the number of home visits required, as patients and carers are encouraged to contact the specialist nurse if any difficulties arise (Barnett, 2003). With improved education, patients are more able to carry out their personal management plan if they develop signs of an exacerbation.

The role of the specialist nurse is very challenging due to the complexity of patients suffering from this chronic disease, but it can also be extremely rewarding in return. The specialist nurse is able to treat the patient using a holistic approach to care as well as forming a therapeutic relationship with the patient, which is very satisfying.

THE ROLE OF THE CONSULTANT RESPIRATORY NURSE

In recent years we have seen a proliferation of new roles within nursing, one of which has been the implementation of the consultant nurse, which was set up by the government in the UK in 1999. The number of consultant respiratory nurses is relatively small compared to other specialities.

This role was developed to keep nurses with clinical skills in practice. The role of the nurse consultant involves the integration of four domains: expert practice; professional leadership and consultancy; education, training and development; and practice and service development involving 50% of working practice directly with patient care. Manley (1997) identifies six core skills and qualities required of a consultant nurse:

- Ability to apply nursing practice to a specific client group, whether as a generalist or a specialist nurse
- Potential leadership skills and a shared strategic vision
- Ability to use research and evaluation approaches that focus on day-to-day issues in daily practice
- To facilitate practice development as well as structural, cultural and practice change
- Provide training and education to enable team members to learn and develop their potential
- To provide expertise from a clinical level in relation to individual patient care and organisational decisions that will enhance the provision of services to meet the needs of the service and patients

Consultant respiratory nurses have the ability and driving force to develop and influence COPD nursing further by responding to the changing needs within the NHS as well as the development of evidence-based and patient-centred practice.

THE ROLE OF THE COMMUNITY MATRON

The government has recently implemented the role of the community matron to tackle chronic disease management. Chronic disease management is being given top priority by the government through a number of policy documents and initiatives, including *Supporting People with Long-Term Conditions* (Department of Health, 2005). It is recognised that the impact of chronic disease on an individual patient's quality of life and the cost to the NHS is enormous. In the past, management of patients with chronic illness has traditionally been reactive, unplanned and episodic (Department of Health, 2005). This often results in emergency hospital admissions, increasing pressure on secondary services. The government has therefore set a target of reducing inpatient emergency bed days by 5%, by March 2008. To help achieve this target it is hoped that by 2007, 3000 community matrons will be in post to help to initiate this plan of care. Community matrons will be responsible for identifying the most vulnerable patients, with highly complex and multiple long-term chronic conditions. They are likely to hold a caseload of 50–80 patients, using a case management approach to identify individual patient needs and implement appropriate care and coordination with members of the multidisciplinary team. Research has shown that case management can improve patients' lives dramatically and also reduce emergency admissions to hospital (Chamberlain-Webber, 2004).

THE ROLE OF THE PRACTICE NURSE

Many practice nurses are now responsible for caring for patients with COPD. Implementation of the NICE guidelines for COPD (National Collaborating Centre for Chronic Conditions, 2004) and the GMS Contract has provided opportunities for practice nurses to provide a better service to patients with COPD as well as enabling them to develop their own skills and knowledge. Such a structured approach should involve the following:

* Development of a COPD register
* Identification of potential patients who may develop COPD (i.e. heavy long-term smokers) by recording spirometry
* Regular patient follow-up clinics to check medication compliance, inhaler technique and symptom control
* Provide patient education on smoking cessation, exercise and diet and self-management
* Encourage the uptake of flu and pneumococcal vaccinations
* Refer to appropriate health specialists/services

As with all health professionals working with patients with COPD, the optimal aims of treatment is to establish an accurate and early diagnosis of COPD and to ensure the patient is receiving optimal drug management therapy to relieve their symptoms and to improve their quality of life.

THE ROLE OF THE PHYSIOTHERAPIST

Physiotherapists are a valuable member of the multidisciplinary team and play a vital role in caring for patients with COPD. They are often requested to help provide specialist advice and support for patients with COPD for the following reasons:

* During an exacerbation of their COPD
* Patients who may have difficulty clearing their chest of secretions
* To help control anxiety and panic attacks that lead to hyperventilation

To help clear secretions often involves teaching the patient the Active Cycle of Breathing Technique (ACBT) using forced expiration to enhance expectoration. Techniques to reduce the work of breathing involve the use of relaxed breathing control, for diaphragmatic breathing control is of benefit to manage panic attacks and breathlessness. Physiotherapists have a vital role to play in pulmonary rehabilitation programmes and in providing support in palliative care. As well as respiratory management the physiotherapist can also provide advice and support for patients with mobility problems.

THE ROLE OF THE OCCUPATIONAL THERAPIST

As emphasised throughout this book, it is essential that patients are regularly asked about their ability to undertake activities of daily living and how their breathlessness affects this. Occupational therapy focuses on helping patients to achieve independence in all areas of their lives and to enhance their quality of life. Assessment tools such as the Manchester Respiratory Activities of Daily Living (MRADL) questionnaire (Yohannes, Greenwood and Connolly, 2002) and the London Chest Activity of Daily Living (LCADL) scale (Garrod, Paul and Wedzicha, 2002) are available and have been validated specifically for patients with COPD. Occupational therapists are also able to provide support and advice to patients recently diagnosed with COPD or patients requiring palliative care, and may also be an active member of the pulmonary rehabilitation team.

THE FUTURE

Until very recently, COPD has had a very poor image and been given low priority within health care. However, this is changing. With the development of various new government policies and initiatives a growing interest is emerging for this long-term chronic illness. The future no longer looks so bleak for our patients who have suffered and struggled so long on their own with little support and understanding, often having been told that nothing more can be done for them. The changes in primary care are moving towards providing a service that will benefit patients in the long term.

A new tier of nurses is emerging who with their expertise will influence patient management and care for the better, providing high-quality evidence-based care. It has been recognised for some time that there is little in the way of medical intervention for these patients. However, there is now some recognition that specialist nurses can make a huge impact on these patients, in terms of symptom control, enhancing quality of life, as well as reducing the number of hospital admissions.

Providing support and understanding to these patients and their carers through education and addressing individual concerns goes a long way to enabling patients to cope with their condition. Supplying patients with individualised care plans/self-management plans enables them to gain control and feel confident, which as a result improves clinical outcomes. Increasing psychosocial and palliative care support where appropriate will also help to increase patient satisfaction and improve care for these patients.

The future for nurses and other health professionals caring for patients with COPD looks both exciting and challenging. There are potentially a lot of changes to implement and to evaluate. Over the next few years an increasing number of community matrons and nurse consultants will be emerging in respiratory nursing. It is hoped they will lead the way with further research on all aspects of COPD. Nurses will learn from this, and in turn this will inevitably help to raise standards of care across both primary and secondary care. Education and continuing professional development is vital for all respiratory nurses in order to enhance skills and knowledge in the field of COPD.

It is hoped that this book will have provided health professionals with a framework and also a resource to provide further knowledge on the special care of patients with COPD, identifying the evidence, support and advice now available to enhance their quality of life.

Glossary

Acidosis. Increased acidity/reduced pH of body fluids. In respiratory acidosis this is due to accumulation of carbon dioxide in the blood.

Acute. Brief, short term and often severe.

Air-trapping. Excess air remaining in the lung at the end of exhalation. This may be due to airway collapse and/or loss of lung elasticity, as in emphysema.

Allergens. Substances that cause an allergic reaction, e.g. dust, pollen, cigarette smoke.

Alpha-1 antitrypsin. A protein produced in the liver, which blocks the action of trypsin and other proteolytic enzymes. An inherited deficiency of alpha-1 antitrypsin, which is associated with early presentation (under 40 years of age) of severe emphysema.

Anticholinergic bronchodilator. A drug that inhibits the action of acetylcholine on the parasympathetic nerve endings which dilates the airways.

Antioxidants. A substance that neutralises oxidants. They occur naturally in foods rich in vitamins C and E and it is thought they may slow down the progression of COPD.

Antiprotease/elastase. This is an enzyme that neutralises protease/elastase, which is an enzyme that is known to destroy lung tissue by digesting elastin, a protein that makes up lung tissue.

Arterial blood gases. An arterial blood sample to measure the amount of oxygen and carbon dioxide dissolved in the plasma. It is measured in kilopascals (kPa).

Asthma. A chronic inflammatory condition of the airways, leading to widespread, variable airway obstruction that is reversible spontaneously or with treatment. Long-standing asthma may over time become unresponsive to treatment.

Atopy. A hereditary predisposition to develop allergic asthma, rhinitis and eczema. It is associated with high levels of antibody IgE.

Auscultation. Listening to the chest with a stethoscope.

Beta-2 agonist bronchodilator. A drug that causes bronchial smooth muscle to relax and allow constricted bronchi to dilate, thereby improving ventilation to the lungs.

'Blue bloater'. A term used to describe an overweight and cyanosed COPD patient, usually at risk of developing cor pulmonale.

Body mass index (BMI). A measure to determine if a person is obese or underweight, defined as weight in kilograms divided by height in metres squared.

Borg scale. A measurement of breathlessness by which the patient quantifies the degree of breathlessness that a particular activity may produce.

Bronchiectasis. Irreversible dilation of the bronchi due to bronchial wall damage, causing chronic cough and excess mucopurulent sputum.

Bronchspasm. Contraction of smooth muscle in the walls of the bronchial tree leading to narrowing of the airway lumen.

Bulla(e). Large cyst-like spaces that compress normal lung tissue.

Chronic bronchitis. The production of sputum that occurs on most days for at least three months in at least two consecutive years.

Chronic obstructive pulmonary disease (COPD). A slowly progressive disorder characterised by airflow obstruction, which does not change markedly over several months.

Cor pulmonale. Right-sided heart failure caused by enlargement of the right ventricle (right ventricular hypertrophy) as a result of primary pulmonary disease.

Corticosteroids. Synthetic drug used in COPD for their anti-inflammatory properties, although their long-term use is controversial.

Cyanosis. Blue/purple coloration of the skin and mucosa usually due to lack of oxygen or hypoxia.

Disability. The extent of a patient's ability to function normally is affected by ill health.

Dynamic airway collapse. The collapse of unsupported airways during forced exhalation.

Dyspnoea. Difficulty in breathing.

Electrocardiograph (ECG). A heart tracing that measures the electrical activity of the heart.

Elastase. An enzyme that digests elastin.

Elastin. Protein that makes up the elastic properties assisting with lung tissue recoil and helps to expel air from the lungs during exhalation.

Emphysema. An irreversible disease of the lungs that is characterised by destruction of the alveolar walls within the lungs.

Eosinophil. White blood cell that is present in the airways of asthmatics.

Exacerbation. A sustained worsening of the individual's symptoms from the usual stable state.

Fibrosis. Scarring and thickening of tissue.

Flow/volume trace. A graph produced by a spirometer in which the flow rate (in litres per second) is on the vertical axis and volume (in litres) on the horizontal axis.

Force expiratory volume (FEV_1). The maximum amount of air that can be expired from the lungs in one second.

Gas exchange. The exchange of waste carbon dioxide produced by the body during respiration of oxygen from the atmosphere.

Guy-rope effect. The support given to the small airways by the elastic walls of the alveoli in the lung tissue.

Haemoptysis. Expectorating of blood from the lungs or bronchial tubes as a result of pulmonary or bronchial haemorrhage.

Health status. A measure of the impact of a disease on a patient's quality of life as well as social and emotional wellbeing.

Hypercapnia. High levels of carbon dioxide in the blood. Levels over 6 kPa are usually considered abnormal.

Hypoxia. Low levels of oxygen in the blood. Levels below 10 kPa are usually considered abnormal.

Hypoxic challenge. A method of assessing the response of a patient to reduced oxygen levels during flight.

Immunoglobulin E (IgE). An antibody. Raised levels of IgE are associated with atopy and allergy.

Inhaled corticosteroids/steroids. Medication available via inhalation using an inhaler device or via a nebuliser.

Lobectomy. Surgical excision of one or more lobes of the lung.

Long-term oxygen therapy (LTOT). Oxygen delivered via a concentrator over a 15-hour period. It improves life expectancy and may improve the quality of life in patients with chronic hypoxia.

Lung volume reduction surgery (LVRS). A surgical technique to remove emphysematous bullae from the lung to improve breathlessness.

Macrophages. White blood cells that are involved in phagocytosis and secretion of cytokines, which attract and activate neutrophils and other inflammatory cells.

Mast cells. White blood cells that release histamine and other inflammatory mediators.

Mucolytics. Drugs that reduce the stickiness of sputum.

Nicotine replacement therapy (NRT). Treatment used to help reduce craving and withdrawal symptoms in individuals attempting to quit smoking. It is available in patches, chewing gum, lozenges, sublingual tablets, inhalator and nasal spray.

Oedema. The accumulation of excess fluid in cells or tissues.

Osteoporosis. Loss of bony tissue, resulting in brittle bones that are liable to fracture.

Oxygen concentrator. An electrically powered machine that delivers oxygen to the patient. It works by removing nitrogen and carbon dioxide from the air via a series of molecular sieves to deliver pure oxygen. It is a cost-effective method of administering long-term oxygen.

Oxygen cost diagram. A tool to measure the degree of disability and breathlessness during activity. The disability is scored against a 10cm line.

Oxygen saturation. This is the percentage of haemoglobin saturated with oxygen measured by using a pulse oximeter. Normal oxygen saturation is over 95%.

Pack years. A method of measuring cigarette smoking history that is calculated by multiplying the number of packs of cigarettes smoked each day by the number of years smoked.

$PaCO_2$. Level of carbon dioxide in the blood.

Peak expiratory flow rate (PEF). Maximum flow rate that can be exhaled over the first 10ms of a forced blow.

'Pink puffer'. A phase used to describe a patient with COPD who is very breathless but has normal arterial blood gases and is not at risk of developing cor pulmonale.

Pleural effusion. An abnormal collection of fluid between the visceral and parietal pleural membranes.

Pneumothorax. A collection of air or gas in the pleural cavity that causes the lung to collapse.

PaO_2. Level of oxygen in the blood.

Polycythaemia. An increase of red blood cells in the blood. It occurs as a result of chronic hypoxia.

Pulmonary hypertension. Raised blood pressure within the blood vessels supplying the lungs.

Pulmonary rehabilitation. A programme of exercises and education for patients with COPD who are disabled due to their breathlessness.

Pulse oximetry. A noninvasive technique used to measure oxygen saturation.

Raynaud's phenomenon. Spasm of the blood vessels of the hands or feet.

Relaxed vital capacity (VC). The capacity of the lungs measured when the patient breathes out steadily.

Respiratory failure. Failure to maintain oxygenation.

Type 1 respiratory failure is hypoxaemia in the absence of hypercapnia.

Type 2 respiratory failure is hypoxaemia with hypercapnia.

Respiratory muscle training. Breathing exercises that are aimed at improving respiratory muscle strength and endurance.

Restrictive lung disease. A disease pattern that causes reduction in lung volumes but a normal FEV_1 / FVC.

Short-burst oxygen. Oxygen therapy prescribed on an 'as-required' basis for the relief of breathlessness or post-exertion.

Shuttle walking test. A method of assessing walking distance in patients with breathlessness. The patient carries out a paced walk between two points 10 m apart dictated by beeps on a tape recording.

Simple bronchitis. Chronic mucus production that is not associated with airflow obstruction.

Spirometry. Measurement of lung volumes and airflow with equipment known as a spirometer.

Theophylline. Oral bronchodilator used in COPD.

Therapeutic range. Dosage range in which a drug exerts a therapeutic effect.

Venturi mask. An oxygen mask that delivers a fixed percentage of oxygen.

Volume/time trace. A graph produced by a spirometer. The volume is plotted on the vertical axis and the time on the horizontal axis.

Wheeze. A sound generated by turbulent airflow through the conducting airways, usually heard on expiration.

References

Agertoft, L. and Pedersen, S. (1994) Effects of long-term treatment with inhaled corticosteroids on growth and pulmonary function in asthmatic children. *Respiratory Medicine*, **88**, 373–81.

Allen, K. (2004) Principles and limitations of pulse oximetry in patient monitoring. *Nursing Times*, **100** (41), 34–7.

Allen, S.C. and Prior, A. (1986) What determines whether an elderly patient can use a metered-dose inhaler correctly? *British Journal of Disease of the Chest*, **80** (1), 45–9.

Ambrosino, N., Montagna, T., Nava, S. *et al.* (1990) Short term effect of intermittent negative pressure ventilation in COPD patients with respiratory failure. *European Respiratory Journal*, **3**, 502–8.

American Thoracic Society (1995) Standards for the diagnosis and care of patients with Chronic Obstructive Pulmonary Disease. *American Journal of Respiratory and Critical Care Medicine*, **152** (5, Pt 2), S77–S121.

American Thoracic Society (1998) International guidelines for the selection of lung transplant candidates. *American Journal of Respiratory and Critical Care Medicine*, **158**, 335–9.

American Thoracic Society (1999) Pulmonary rehabilitation. *American Journal of Respiratory and Critical Care Medicine*, **159** (5), 1666–82.

Argenziano, M., Thomashow, B., Jellen, P.A. *et al.* (1997) Functional comparison of unilateral versus bilateral lung volume reduction surgery. *Annals of Thoracic Surgery*, **64**, 321–6.

ASH (2005) *Basic Facts: One. Smoking Statistics*, Action on Smoking and Health, January 2005; www.ash.org.uk (accessed September 2005).

Association of Respiratory Technicians and Physiologists/British Thoracic Society (1994) Guidelines for the measurement of respiratory function. *Respiratory Medicine*, **88** (3), 165–94.

Barker, D.J., Goffrey, K.M., Fall, C. *et al.* (1991) Relation of birth weight and childhood respiratory infection to adult lung function and death from chronic obstructive airways disease. *British Medical Journal*, **303**, 671–5.

Barley, E.A., Quirk, F.H. and Jones, P.W. (1998) Asthma health status measurement in clinical practice: validity of a new short and simple instrument. *Respiratory Medicine*, **92** (10), 1207–14.

Barnett, M. (2003) A nurse-led community scheme for managing patients with COPD. *Professional Nurse*, **19** (2); 93–6.

Barnes, P.J. (1999) *Managing Chronic Obstructive Pulmonary Disease*, Science Press Ltd, London.

Beck, A.T. (1980) *Beck Anxiety Inventory*, Harcourt Brace Jovanovich, Inc., San Antonio, California.

Beck, A.T., Steer, R.A. and Brown, G.K. (1986) *Beck Depression Inventory*, Harcourt Brace Jovanovich, Inc., San Antonio, California.

Bellamy, D. and Booker, R. (2003) *Chronic Obstructive Pulmonary Disease in Primary Care*, Class Publishing, London.

Benson, H.A. and Prankered, R.J. (1998) Optimisation of drug delivery – pulmonary drug delivery. *Australian Journal of Hospital Pharmacy*, **28**, 18–23.

Bergner, M. (1988) Measurement of health status. *Medical Care*, **5** (23), 696–704.

Billings, J.A. (2000) Palliative care. *British Medical Journal*, **321**, 555–8.

Biskobing, D.M. (2002) COPD and osteoporosis. *Chest*, **121**, 609–10.

Booker, R. (2004a) Pharmacology of bronchodilators. *Nursing Times*, **100** (6), 54–9.

Booker, R. (2004b) Pulse oximetry in primary care. *The Airways Journal*, **2** (3), 146–8.

Booker, R. (2005) Chronic obstructive pulmonary disease and the NICE guideline. *Nursing Standard*, **19** (22), 43–52.

Borg, G. (1982) Psychophysical basis of perceived exertion. *Medicine and Science in Sports and Exercise*, **14** (5), 377–81.

Bourke, S.J. (2003) *Respiratory Medicine*, Blackwell Publishing Ltd, Oxford.

Bourke, S.J. and Brewis, R. (1998) *Respiratory Medicine*, Blackwell Science, Oxford.

Boyars, M.C. (1988) COPD in the ambulatory elderly: management update. *Geriatrics*, **43**, 29–40.

Braun, S.R., McKenzie, W.N., Copeland, C. *et al.* (1989) A comparison of the effect of Ipratropium and Albuterol in the treatment of chronic airways disease. *Archives of Internal Medicine*, **149**, 544–7.

Bredin, M. (1998) Multicentre randomised controlled trail of a nursing intervention for breathlessness in patients with lung cancer. *Palliative Medicine*, **12** (6), 470.

British Lung Foundation and British Thoracic Society (2003) *Pulmonary Rehabilitation Survey*, British Lung Foundation, London.

British National Formulary (2005) *British National Formulary No. 49*, British Medical Association and the Royal Pharmaceutical Society of Great Britain, London.

British Thoracic Society (1997a) Current best practice for nebuliser treatment. *Thorax*, **52** (Suppl. 2), S1–S106.

British Thoracic Society (1997b) COPD guidelines for the management of chronic obstructive pulmonary disease. *Thorax*, **52** (Suppl. 5), S1–S28.

British Thoracic Society (2002a) Non-invasive ventilation in acute respiratory failure. *Thorax*, **57** (3), 192–211.

British Thoracic Society (2002b) *The Burden of Lung Disease*, British Thoracic Society, London.

Brown, R. (2004) Drug delivery systems 2. Pulmonary and parental formulations. *Airways Journal*, **2** (1), 43–6.

Brusasco, V., Hodder, R., Miravitlles, M. *et al.* (2003) Health outcomes following treatment for six months with once daily tiotropium compared with twice daily salmeterol in patients with COPD. *Thorax*, **58**, 399–404.

Burge, P.S. (1994) Occupation and chronic obstructive pulmonary disease. *European Respiratory Journal*, **7**, 1032–4.

Burge, P.S., Calverley, P.M.A., Jones, P.W. *et al.* (2000) Randomised, double-blind, placebo-controlled study of fluticasone propionate in patients with moderate to severe chronic obstructive pulmonary disease: the Isolde trial. *British Medical Journal*, **320**, 1297–303.

Calverley, P., Pauwels, R., Vestbo, J. *et al.* (2003) Combined salmeterol and fluticasone in the treatment of chronic obstructive pulmonary disease: a randomised controlled trial. *The Lancet*, **361**, 449–56.

Carroll, P. (1997) Pulse oximetry at your fingertips. *Registered Nurse*, **60** (2), 22–7.

Casaburi, R., Mahler, D.A., Jones, P.W. *et al.* (2002) A long-term evaluation of one-daily inhaled tiotropium in chronic obstructive pulmonary disease. *European Respiratory Journal*, **19**, 217–24.

Chamberlain-Webber, J. (2004) Tackling chronic disease. *Professional Nurse*, **20** (4), 14–18.

Collins, C. (2003) Nutrition and the COPD patient. *The Airways Journal*, **1**, 94–7.

Connolly, M.J. (1995) Inhaler technique of elderly patients: comparison of metered-dose inhalers and large volume spacer devices. *Age Ageing*, **24** (3), 190–2.

Coombs, M. (2001) Making sense of arterial blood gases. *Nursing Times*, **97** (27), 36–8.

Corner, J. and Driscoll, M. (1999) Development of a breathlessness assessment guide for use in palliative care. *Palliative Medicine*, **13**, 375–84.

Corris, P.A. (1999) Lung transplanation for chronic obstructive pulmonary disease: an exercise in quality rather than quantity? *Thorax*, **54** (Suppl. 2), S24–S27.

Cotton, M.M., Bucknall, C.E., Dragg, K.D. *et al.* (2000) Early discharge for patients with exacerbations of chronic obstructive pulmonary disease: a randomised controlled trial. *Thorax*, **55**, 902–6.

Criner, G., Cordova, F.C., Leyenson, V. *et al.* (1998) Effect of lung volume reduction surgery on diaphragm strength. *American Journal of Respiratory and Critical Care Medicine*, **157**, 1578–85.

Crockett, A. (2000) *Managing Chronic Obstructive Pulmonary Disease in Primary Care*, Blackwell-Science Ltd, Oxford.

Croghan, E. (2005) Prescribing for a successful quit. *Independent Nurse*, 10 January 2005, 20–1.

Davis, C. (1997) The ABC of palliative care: breathlessness, cough and other respiratory symptoms. *British Medical Journal*, **315**, 931–4.

Davis, L., Wilkinson, M., Bonner, S. *et al.* (2000) 'Hospital at home' verses hospital care in patients with exacerbations of chronic obstructive pulmonary disease: prospective randomised controlled trial. *British Medical Journal*, **321**, 1265–8.

Dennis, R.J., Maldonado, D., Norman, S. *et al.* (1996) Wood smoke exposure and risk for obstructive airways disease among women. *Chest*, **109**, 115–19.

Department of Health (1998) *Smoking Kills: A White Paper on Tobacco*, The Stationery Office, London.

Department of Health (1999) *Domiciliary Oxygen Therapy Services: Clinical Guidelines and Advice for Prescribers*, Department of Health, London.

Department of Health (2003) Continuing success of NHS services to help smokers quit, Press Release 0276.

Department of Health (2004a) *A Modernised, Integrated Domiciliary Oxygen Service. Proposals for New Guidelines for the Use of Domiciliary Oxygen*, Department of Health, London; www.dh.gov.uk/policyand guidance/medicinespharmacy and industry/prescriptions/fs/en.

Department of Health (2004b) *Choosing Health: Making Healthy Choices Easier*, The Stationery Office, London.

Department of Health (2005) *Supporting People with Long-Term Conditions*, Department of Health, London.

Donaldson, G.C., Seemungal, T.A., Wedzicha, J.A. *et al.* (2002) Relationship between exacerbation frequency and lung decline in chronic obstructive pulmonary disease. *Thorax*, **57**, 847–52.

Edmonds, P. (2001) A comparison of the palliative care needs of patients dying from chronic respiratory disease and lung cancer. *Palliative Medicine*, **15** (4), 287–95.

Esmond, G. (2001) *Respiratory Nursing*, Bailliere Tindall, London.

Eve, A., Smith, A.M. and Tebbit, P. (1997) Hospice and palliative care in the UK 1994–5. *Palliative Medicine*, **11**, 31–43.

Fehrenbach, C. (2005) Initiatives to improve outcomes for chronic obstructive pulmonary disease. *Professional Nurse*, **20** (6), 43–5.

Fletcher, C.M. and Peto, R. (1977) The natural history of chronic flow obstruction. *British Medical Journal*, **1**, 1645–8.

Fletcher, C.M., Elmes, P.C., Fairburn, M.B. *et al.* (1959) The significance of respiratory symptoms and the diagnosis of chronic bronchitis in a working population. *British Medical Journal*, **2**, 257–66.

Gaber, K.A., Barnett, M., Planchant, Y. *et al.* (2004) Attitudes of 100 patients with chronic obstructive pulmonary disease to artificial ventilation and cardiopulmonary resuscitation. *Palliative Medicine*, **18**, 626–9.

Gagnon, L., Boulet, L.P., Brown, J. *et al.* (1997) Influences on inhaled corticosteroids and dietary intake on bone density and metabolism in patients with moderate to severe asthma. *Journal of American Diet Association*, **97**, 1401–6.

Garrod, R., Paul, E.A. and Wedzicha, J.A. (2002) An evaluation of the reliability and sensitivity of the London Chest Activity of Daily Living Scale (LCADL). *Respiratory Medicine*, **96**, 725–30.

Global Initiative for Chronic Obstructive Lung Disease (2003) Global strategy for the diagnosis, management, and prevention of Chronic Obstructive Pulmonary Disease. NHLBI/WHO Workshop Report, National Institutes of Health.

Godfrey, K. (2004) New guidance on long-term oxygen therapy management and delivery. *Nursing Times*, **100** (38), 57.

Gordois, A. and Gibbons, D. (2002) The cost-effectiveness of outreach respiratory care for COPD patients. *Professional Nurse*, **17** (8), 504–7.

Gore, J.M., Brophy, C.J. and Greenstone, M.A. (2000) How well do we care for patients with end stage chronic obstructive pulmonary disease (COPD)? A comparison of palliative care and quality of life in COPD and lung cancer. *Thorax*, **55**, 1000–6.

Gorse, G.J., Otto, E.E., Daughaday, C.C. *et al.* (1997) Influenza virus vaccination of patients with chronic lung disease. *Chest*, **112** (5), 1221–33.

Gravil, J.H., Al-Rawas, O.A., Cotton, M.M. *et al.* (1999) Home treatment of COPD exacerbations. *Thorax*, **54** (Suppl. 2), S8–S13.

Gregory, S. and Bason, A. (2003) Smoking cessation: is it worth the effort? *Update*, **66** (5), 283–7.

Guyatt, G.H., Berman, L.B., Townsend, M. *et al.* (1987) A measure of quality of life for clinical trials in chronic lung disease. *Thorax*, **42** (10), 773–8.

Haahtela, T., Jarvinen, M., Kava, T. *et al.* (1991) Comparison of a beta 2-agonist, terbutaline, with an inhaled corticosteroid, budesonide, in newly detected asthma. *New England Journal of Medicine*, **325**, 388–92.

Halpin, D.M. (2001) *COPD Rapid Reference*, Harcourt Publishers Ltd, London.

Halpin, D.M. (2003) *Your Questions Answered: COPD*, Churchill Livingstone, London.

Halpin, D.M. (2004) Bronchodilators in COPD: the long and short of it. *The Airways Journal,* **2** (1), 30–2.

Hampson, N. (1998) Pulse oximetry in severe carbon monoxide posing. *Chest,* **114** (4), 1036–41.

Hansel, T.T. and Barnes, P.J. (2004) *An Atlas of Chronic Obstructive Pulmonary Disease (COPD),* Parthenon Publishing Group, London.

Hendrick, D.J. (1996) Occupation and chronic obstructive pulmonary disease (COPD). *Thorax,* **51**, 947–55.

Heslop, K. and Rao, S. (2003) Cognitive behavioural therapy for patients with respiratory disease. *The Airways Journal,* **1**, 139–41.

Higenbottam, T. (1997) Key issues in nebulised drug delivery in adults. *European Respiratory Review,* **51** (Suppl. 7), 378–9.

Holland, K., Jenkins, J., Soloman, K. *et al.* (2003) *Applying the Roper, Logan, Tierney Model in Practice,* Churchill Livingstone, London.

Hubbard, R.B., Smith, C.J., Smeeth, L. *et al.* (2002) Inhaled corticosteroids and hip fracture: a population-based case-control study. *American Journal of Respiratory and Critical Care Medicine,* **166**, 1563–6.

Jeffery, P.K. (1998) Structural and inflammatory changes in COPD: a comparison with asthma. *Thorax,* **53**, 129–36.

Jenkins, S.C., Heaton, R.W. and Fulton, T.J. (1987) Comparison of a domiciliary nebulised salbutamol and salbutamol from a metered dose inhaler in stable chronic airflow limitation. *Chest,* **91**, 804–7.

Johns, D.P. and Pierce, R. (2003) *Pocket Guide to Spirometry,* McGraw-Hill Australia Pty Ltd.

Johnson, M.K. and Stevenson, R.D. (2002) Management of acute exacerbation of chronic obstructive pulmonary disease: are we ignoring the evidence? *Thorax,* **57** (Suppl. 11), 15–23.

Johnson, M.K., Smith, R.P., Mirison, D. *et al.* (2000) Large bullae in marijuana smokers. *Thorax,* **55**, 340–2.

Jones, P. (2001) *Assessing Treatment Outcomes in COPD,* Synergy Medical Education, London.

Jones, P.W. and Bosh, T.K. (1997) Quality of life changes in COPD patients treated with salmeterol. *American Journal of Respiratory and Critical Care Medicine,* **155** (4), 1283–9.

Jones, P.W., Quirk, F.H., Baveystock, C.M. *et al.* (1992) A self-complete measure for chronic airflow limitation: the St George's Respiratory Questionnaire. *American Review of Respiratory Disease,* **145**, 1321–7.

Jones, R.C.M., Hyland, M.E., Hanney, K. *et al.* (2004) A qualitative study of compliance with medication and lifestyle modification in chronic obstructive pulmonary disease (COPD). *Primary Care Respiratory Journal,* **13**, 149–54.

Keatings, V.M., Jatakanon, A., Wordell, Y.M. *et al.* (1997) Effects of inhaled and oral glucocorticoids on inflammatory indices in asthma and COPD. *American Journal of Respiratory and Critical Care Medicine*, **155**, 542–8.

Kroll, J.D. (2001) Concerns and needs for research in herbal supplement. Pharmacotherapy and safety. *Journal of Herbal Pharmacotherapy*, **1** (2), 3–23.

Kunik, M.E., Braun, V., Stanleyt, M.A. *et al.* (2001) One-session cognitive behavioural therapy for elderly patients with chronic obstructive pulmonary disease. *Psychol. Medicine*, **31**, 717–23.

Lacasse, Y., Wong, E., Guyatt, G.H. *et al.* (1996) Meta-analysis of respiratory rehabilitation in chronic obstructive pulmonary disease. *Lancet*, **348**, 1115–19.

Landbo, C., Prescott, E., Lange, P. *et al.* (1999) Prognostic value of nutritional status in chronic obstructive pulmonary disease. *American Journal of Respiratory and Critical Care Medicine*, **160**, 1856–61.

Law, C. (2001) Sexual health and the respiratory patient. *Nursing Times Plus Suppl.*, **97** (12), 11–13.

Lewith, G.T. (1998) Respiratory illness: a complementary perspective. *Thorax*, **53** (10), 898–904.

Lisansky, D.P. and Clough, D.H. (1996) A cognitive-behavioral self-help educational program for patients with COPD. A pilot study. *Psychotherapy Psychom.*, **65**, 97–101.

Lung Health Study Research Group (2000) Effect of inhaled triamcinolone on the decline of pulmonary function in COPD. *New England Journal of Medicine*, **343**, 1902–9.

McEvoy, C.E. and Niewoehner, D.E. (1997) Adverse effects of corticosteroid therapy for COPD. A critical review. *Chest*, **3**, 732–43.

McGavin, C.R., Artvinli, M. and Naoe, H. (1978) Dyspnoea, disability and distance walked: a comparison of estimates of exercise performance in respiratory disease. *British Medical Journal*, **2**, 241–3.

McLauchlan, L. (2002) Supplementary oxygen therapy in the community. *Nursing Times Plus Suppl.*, **98** (40), 50–2.

McLoughlin, C. (2005) Nicotine replacement. *Professional Nurse*, **20** (7), 50–1.

Mahler, D.A., Donohue, J.F., Barbee, R.A. *et al.* (1999) Efficacy of salmeterol in the treatment of COPD. *Chest*, **115**, 957–65.

Manley, K. (1997) A conceptual framework for advanced practice. *Journal of Clinical Nursing*, **6** (3), 179–90.

Masi, M.A., Hanley, J.A., Ernest, P. *et al.* (1988) Environmental exposure to tobacco smoke and lung function in young adults. *American Review of Respiratory Disorders*, **138**, 296–9.

Matthay, R.A. and Mahler, D.A. (1986) Theophylline improves global cardiac function and reduces dyspnea in chronic obstructive pulmonary disease. *Journal of Allergy and Clinical Immunology*, **78**, 793–9.

Matthews, H., Browne, P., Sawyer, S. *et al.* (2001) Lifesaver or life sentence? *Nursing Times*, **97** (34), 46–8.

Medical Research Council (1981) Report of the Oxygen Working Party. Long-term domiciliary oxygen therapy in chronic hypoxic cor pulmonale complicating chronic bronchitis and emphysema. *Lancet*, **1**, 681–6.

Meecham-Jones, D.J., Paul, E.A., Jones, P.W. *et al.* (1995) Nasal pressure support ventilation plus oxygen compared with oxygen therapy alone in hypercapnic COPD. *American Journal of Respiratory and Critical Care Medicine*, **152**, 538–44.

Morgan, W.J. (1998) Maternal smoking and infants lung function. Further evidence for an *in utero* effect. *American Journal of Respiratory and Critical Care Medicine*, **158**, 689–90.

Morgan, M. (1999) The prediction of benefit from pulmonary rehabilitation: setting, training intensity and the effect of selection by disability. *Thorax*, **54** (Suppl. 2), S3–S7.

Murciano, D., Aubier, M., Lecocguic, Y. *et al.* (1984) Effect of theophylline on diaphragmatic strength and fatigue in patients with chronic obstructive pulmonary disease. *New England Journal of Medicine*, **311**, 349–53.

Murray, C.J. and Lopez, A.D. (1996) Evidence-based health policy: lessons from the global burden of disease study. *Science*, **274**, 740–3.

National Collaborating Centre for Chronic Conditions (2004) Chronic Obstructive Pulmonary Disease. National clinical guideline on management of Chronic Obstructive Pulmonary Disease in adults in primary and secondary care. *Thorax*, **59** (Suppl. 1), 1–232.

National Institute for Clinical Excellence (2002) *Guidance on the Use of Nicotine Replacement Therapy (NRT) and Bupropion for Smoking Cessation. Technology Appraisal Guidance No. 39*, NICE, London.

Nichol, K.L., Baken, L., Wuorenma, J. *et al.* (1999) The health and economic benefits associated with pneumococcal vaccination of elderly persons with chronic lung disease. *Archives of Internal Medicine*, **159**, 2437–42.

Niziol, C. (2004) Respiratory care in community settings. *Nursing Standard*, **6** (19), 41–5.

Nocturnal Oxygen Therapy Trial (1980) Continuous or nocturnal oxygen therapy in hypoxemic chronic obstructive lung disease: a clinical trial. *Annals of Internal Medicine*, **93**, 391–8.

Noseda, A., Capreiaux, J.P. and Schmerber, J. (1992) Dyspnoea assessed by visual analogue scale in patients with obstructive lung disease during progressive and high-intensity exercise. *Thorax*, **47** (5), 363–8.

O'Brien, T., Welsh, J. and Dunn, F.G. (1998) ABC of palliative care: non-malignant conditions. *British Medical Journal*, **316**, 286–9.

O'Neill, B. and Rodway, A. (1998) ABC of palliative care: care in the community. *British Medical Journal*, **316**, 373–7.

Orem, D. (1971) *Nursing: Concepts of Practice*, McGraw-Hill, New York.

Osman, I.M., Gedden, D.J., Friend, J.A. *et al.* (1997) Quality of life and hospital readmission in patients with chronic obstructive pulmonary disease. *Thorax*, **52**, 67–71.

Pauwels, R.A., Lofdani, C., Laitinen, L.A. *et al.* (1999) Long-term treatment with inhaled budesonide in persons with mild chronic obstructive pulmonary disease who continue smoking. *New England Journal of Medicine*, **340**, 1948–53.

Pepin, K.L. (1996) Long-term oxygen therapy at home. *Chest*, **109** (5), 1144–50.

Percival, J. (2002) Strategies for smoking cessation. *Nursing Times Plus Suppl.*, **98** (40), 66–7.

Plant, P.K. and Elliott, M.W. (2003) Management of ventilatory failure in COPD. *Thorax*, **58**, 537–42.

Poole, P. and Black, P. (2001) Oral mucolytic drugs for exacerbations of chronic obstructive pulmonary disease: systematic review. *British Medical Journal*, **322** (7297), 1271–4.

Quanjer, G.J., Tammeling, J.E., Cotes, O.F. *et al.* (1993) Lung volumes and forced ventilatory flows, Report of the Working Party: Standardization of lung function tests, European Community for Steel and Coal. *European Respiratory Society*, **6** (Suppl. 16), 4–40.

Rasmussen, F., Taylor, D.R., Flannery, E.M. *et al.* (2002) Risk factors for airway remodelling in asthma manifested by a low post-bronchodilator FEV_1/vital capacity ration: a longitudinal population study from childhood to adulthood. *American Journal of Respiratory and Critical Care Medicine*, **165**, 1467–8.

Reed, C.E. (1999) The natural history of asthma in adults: the problem of irreversibility. *Journal of Allergy and Clinical Immunology*, **103**, 539–47.

Respiratory Alliance (2003) *Bridging the Gap: Commissioning and Delivering High-Quality Integrated Respiratory Health Care*, Direct Publishing Solutions, Cookham, Berkshire.

Riches, A. (2003) Non-invasive ventilation and COPD. *Nursing Times*, **99** (20), 49.

Roberts, C.M., Lowe, D., Bucknall, C.E. *et al.* (2002) Clinical audit indicators of outcome following admission to hospital with acute exacerbation of chronic obstructive pulmonary disease. *Thorax*, **57**, 137–41.

Rodriguez-Roisin, R. (2000) Towards a consensus definition for COPD exacerbations. *Chest*, **117**, 398S–401S.

Rogers, M. (1970) *An Introduction to the Theoretical Basis of Nursing*, F.A. Davis, Philadelphia.

Roper, N., Logan, W.W. and Tierney, A.J. (1996) *The Elements of Nursing*, 4th edn, Churchill Livingstone, Edinburgh.

Roper, N., Logan, W.W. and Tierney, A.J. (2000) *The Roper Logan Tierney Model of Nursing Based on Activities of Living*, Churchill Livingstone, Edinburgh.

Roper, N., Logan, W.W. and Tierney, A.J. (2001) *The Elements of Nursing. A Model for Nursing Based on a Model of Living*, Churchill Livingstone, Edinburgh.

Rose, K. (1995) Palliative care: the nurse's role. *Nursing Standard*, **10** (11), 38–44.

Roy, C. (1970) Adaptation: a conceptual framework for nursing. *Nursing Outlook*, **18** (3), 42–5.

Royal College of Physicians (1999) *Domiciliary Oxygen Therapy Services*, Royal College of Physicians, London, pp. S77–S121.

Royal College of Physicians (2000) *Nicotine Addiction in Britain. A Report of the Tobacco Advisory Group of the Royal College of Physicians*, Royal College of Physicians, London.

Sauerwein, H.P. and Romijn, J.A. (1999) More consideration to dietary protein in the nutrition of chronically ill adults with a tendency to weight loss. *Ned Tijdschr Geneeskd*, **143**, 886–9; also in Collins, C. (2003) Nutrition and the COPD patient. *The Airways Journal*, **1**, 94–7.

Scholey, A. and Moss, M. (2005) Nicotine and caffeine; available at www.psychology.unn.ac.uk/PY116/HPnicotine (accessed February 2005).

Schols, A. and Wouters, E.F. (2000) Nutritional abnormalities and supplementation in chronic obstructive pulmonary disease. *Clinical Chest Medicine*, **21**, 753–62.

Schols, A.M., Slangen, J., Volovics, L. *et al.* (1998) Weight loss is a reversible factor in the prognosis of chronic obstructive pulmonary disease. *American Journal of Respiratory and Critical Care Medicine*, **157**, 1791–7.

Sciurba, F.C., Rogers, R.M., Keenan, R.J. *et al.* (1996) Improvement in pulmonary function and elastic recoil after lung-reduction surgery for diffuse emphysema. *New England Journal of Medicine*, **334**, 1095–9.

Sharpe, D.S., Rodriguez, B.L., Shahar, E. *et al.* (1994) Fish consumption may limit the damage of smoking on the lung. *American Journal of Respiratory and Critical Care Medicine*, **150**, 983–7.

Siafakas, N.M., Vermeire, P., Pride, N.B. *et al.* (1995) Optimal assessment and management of chronic obstructive pulmonary disease (COPD). The European Respiratory Society Task Force. *European Respiratory Journal*, **8** (8), 1398–420.

Small, S. and Lamb, M. (1999) Fatigue in chronic illness: the experience of individuals with COPD and with asthma. *Journal of Advanced Nursing*, **30** (2), 469–78.

Snaith, R.P. and Zigmond, A.S. (1994) *Hospital Anxiety and Depression Scale*, NFER-Nelson Publishing Company, Windsor.

Social Trends (1995) HMSO, London.

Stick, S. (2000) The contribution of airway development to paediatric and adult lung disease. *Thorax*, **55**, 587–94.

Strachan, D.P., Seagroatt, V., Cook, D.G. *et al.* (1994) Chest illness in infancy and chronic respiratory disease in later life: an analysis by month of birth. *International Journal of Epidemiology*, **23**, 1060–8.

Stratton, K., Shetty, P., Wallace, R. and Bondurant, S. (2001) *Clearing the Smoke: Assessing the Science Base for Tobacco Harm Reduction*, National Academy Press, Washington, DC.

Sutherland, E.R. and Cherniack, R.M. (2004) Management of chronic obstructive pulmonary disease. *New England Journal of Medicine*, **350**, 2689–97.

Szafranski, W., Cukier, A., Ramirez, A. *et al.* (2003) Efficacy and safety of budesonide/formoterol in the management of chronic obstructive pulmonary disease. *European Respiratory Journal*, **21**, 74–81.

Tashkin, D.P., Altose, M.D., Connett, J.E. *et al.* (1996) Methacholine reactivity predicts changes in lung function over time in smokers with early chronic obstructive pulmonary disease. The Lung Health Study Research Group. *American Journal of Respiratory and Critical Care Medicine*, **153** (6 Pt 1), 1802–11.

Tashkin, D.P., Simmons, M.S., Sherrill, D.L. *et al.* (1997) Heavy habitual marijuana smoking does not cause an accelerated decline in FEV_1 with age. *American Journal of Respiratory and Critical Care Medicine*, **155**, 141–8.

Thompson, G. (2002) Prescribing of long-term oxygen therapy. *Pharmaceutical Journal*, **268**, 619–20.

Trendall, J. (2000) Concept analysis: chronic fatigue. *Journal of Advanced Nursing*, **32** (5), 1126–31.

Trendall, J. (2001) Assessing fatigue in patients with COPD. *Professional Nurse*, **16** (7), 1217–20.

Trulock, E.P. (1998) Lung transplantation for COPD. *Chest*, **113** (4), 269S–276S.

Twycross, R. (1999) *Introducing Palliative Care*, Radcliff Medical Press Ltd, Abingdon, Oxfordshire.

Ulrik, C.S. and Lange, P. (1994) Decline of lung function in adults with bronchial asthma. *American Journal of Respiratory and Clinical Care Medicine*, **50**, 629–34.

Van Der Molen, T., Willemse, B.W., Schokker, S. *et al.* (2003) Development, validity and responsiveness of the clinical COPD questionnaire. *Health Quality Life Outcomes*, **28** (1), 880–7.

Van Grunsven, P.M., Van Schayck, C.P., Derenne, J.P. *et al.* (1999) Long term effects of inhaled corticosteroids in chronic obstructive pulmonary disease: a meta-analysis. *Thorax*, **54**, 7–14.

Van Hoozen, B.E. and Cross, C.E. (1997) Marijuana respiratory tract effects. *Clinical Review of Allergy Immunology*, **15**, 243–69.

Vassallo, R. and Lipsky, J.J. (1998) Theophylline: recent advances in the understanding of its mode of action and uses in clinical practice. *Mayo Clinic Proceedings*, **73**, 346–54.

Vestbo, J., Sorensen, T., Lange, P. *et al.* (1999) Long-term effects of inhaled budesonide in mild and moderate chronic obstructive pulmonary disease: a randomised controlled trial. *Lancet*, **353**, 1819–23.

Vickers, A. (2000) Complementary medicine. *British Medical Journal*, **321**, 683–6.

Vilagoftis, H., Schwingshackl, A., Milne, C.D. *et al.* (2000) Protease-activated receptor-2-mediated matrix metalloproteinase-9 release from airway epithelial cells. *Journal of Allergy Clinical Immunology*, **106**, 537–45.

Vincken, W., van Noord, J.A., Greefhorst, A.P.M. *et al.* (2002) Improved health outcomes in patients with COPD during 1 years treatment with tiopropium. *European Respiratory Journal*, **19**, 209–16.

Watson, L., Margetts, B., Howarth, P. *et al.* (2002) The association between diet and chronic obstructive pulmonary disease in subjects selected from general practice. *European Respiratory Journal*, **20**, 313–8.

Watson, M., Lucus, C., Hoy, A. *et al.* (2005) *Oxford Handbook of Palliative Care*, Oxford University Press, Oxford.

Wedzicha, J.A. (2002) Exacerbations: etiology and pathophysiologic mechanisms. *Chest*, **121** (5), 136S–141S.

Wegg, J.G. and Hass, F.C. (1998) Long-term oxygen therapy for COPD. *Postgraduate Medicine*, **103** (4), 1.

Whitehead, N. (2003) Herbal remedies: integration into conventional medicine. *Nursing Times*, **99** (43), 30–3.

Wisser, W., Tschernko, E., Senbaklavaci, O. *et al.* (1997) Functional improvement after volume reduction: sternotomy versus videoendoscopic approach. *Annals of Thoracic Surgery*, **63**, 822–7.

Woo, K. (2000) A pilot study to examine the relationships of dyspnoea, physical activity and fatigue in patients with chronic obstructive pulmonary disease. *Journal of Clinical Nursing*, **9** (4), 526–33.

Woodrow, P. (2000) *Intensive Care Nursing*, Routledge, London.

Wookcock, A.A., Grodd, E.R. and Geddes, D.M. (1981) Oxygen relieves breathlessness in 'pink puffers'. *Lancet*, **1**, 907–9.

World Health Organisation (2002) WHO definition of palliative care; www.int/dsa.justpub/cpl/htm (accessed 28/6/05).

Yohannes, A.M., Greenwood, Y.A. and Connolly, M.J. (2002) Reliability of the Manchester respiratory activities of daily living questionnaire as a good postal questionnaire. *Age Ageing*, **31**, 335–8.

Young, J., Fry-Smith, A. and Hyde, C. (1999) Lung volume reduction surgery for chronic obstructive pulmonary disease with underlying severe emphysema. *Thorax*, **54**, 779–89.

Ziment, I. (1987) Theophylline and mucociliary clearance. *Chest*, **92**, 38S–43S.

Useful Addresses

Association of Respiratory Technology and Physiology

ARTP Administration
Suite 4 Sovereign House
Gate Lane
Boldmere
Birmingham B73 5TT
Tel: 0845 2263062
Website: www.arpt.org.uk

Action on Smoking and Health (ASH)

102 Clifton Street
London EC2A 4HW
Tel: 020 7739 5902
Website: www.ash.org.uk/

Breathe Easy Club

British Lung Foundation
73–75 Goswell Road
London EC1V 7ER
Tel: 020 7688 5555
Website: www.lunguk.org

British Homeopathic Association

Hahneman House
29 Park Street West
Luton LU1 3BE
Tel: 0870 4443950
Website: www.trustomeopathy.org

British Lung Foundation

British Lung Foundation
73–75 Goswell Road
London EC1V 7ER
Tel: 020 7688 5555
Website: www.britishlungfoundation.com

British Medical Acupuncture Society

BMAS House
3 Winnington Court
Northwich
Cheshire CW8 1AQ
Tel: 01606 786782
Website: www.medical-acupuncture.co.uk

British Thoracic Society

17 Doughty Street
London WC1N 2PL
Tel: 020 7831 8778
Website: www.brit-thoracic.org.uk

Care Direct

Freephone: 0800 444000
Website: www.caredirect.gov.uk
Note: only available in Southwest England. A phone advice service available
for a person over 60 regarding benefits, home care packages and liaison with
relevant agencies.

Carers UK

20–25 Glasshouse Yard
London EC1A 4JT
Helpline: 0808 808 7777
Tel: 020 7490 8818
Website: www.carersonline.org.uk

Complementary Medical Association

67 Eagle Heights
The Falcons, Bramlands Close
London SW11 2LJ
Helpline: 0845 129 8434
Tel: 01424 438 801
Website: www.the-cma.org.uk

Crossroads Caring for Carers

10 Regent Place
Rugby
Warwickshire CV21 2PN
Helpline: 0845 450 0350
Tel: 01788 573 653
Website: www.crossroads.org.uk

Expert Patient Programme

Tel: 0845 606 6040
Website: www.expertpatients.nhs.uk

General Practice Airways Group (GPIAG)

8th floor, Edgbaston House
3 Duchess Place
Birmingham B16 8NH
Tel: 0121 454 8219
Website: www.gpiag.org

National Respiratory Training Centre

The Athenaeum
10 Church Street
Warwick CV34 4AB
Tel: 01926 493313
Website: www.nrtc.org.uk

Quit (smoking quit lines)

Victory House
Tottenham Court Road
London W1P 0HA
Tel: 020 7388 5775
QUITLINE: 0800 00 22 00
Website: http://healthnet.org.uk/quit/

Respiratory Education Resources Centre

University Hospital
University Clinical Departments
Lower Lane
Aintree
Liverpool L9 7AL
Tel: 0151 529 2598
Website: www.respiratoryerc.com

Royal College of Physicians of Edinburgh

9 Queen Street
Edinburgh EH2 1JQ
Tel: 0131 225 7324
Website: www.rcpe.ac.uk/

DRUG COMPANIES

Allen & Hanburys Ltd

Stockley Park West
Uxbridge
Middlesex UB11 1BT
Tel: 0800 221 441
Website: www.gsk.com

AstraZeneca

AstraZeneca UK Ltd
Horizon Place
600 Capability Green
Luton
Bedfordshire LU1 3LU
Tel: 0800 7830 033
Website: www.medical.informationgb@astraZeneca.com

Boehringer Ingelheim

Boehringer Ingelheim Ltd
Ellesfield Ave
Bracknell
Berkshire RG12 8YS
Tel: 01344 424 600
Website: www.medinfo@bra.boehringer-ingelheim.com

3M Health Care Ltd

3M House
Morley Street
Loughborough
Leicestershire LE11 1EP
Tel: 01509 611611
Website: 3mhealthcare.co.uk

MANUFACTURERS

Clement Clarke International Ltd

Unit A
Cartel Business Estate
Edinburgh Way
Harlow
Essex CM20 2TT
Tel: 01279 414969
Website: www.clement-clarke.com

MicroMedical

Quayside
Chatham Maritime
Chatham
Kent ME4 4QY
Tel: 01634 893500
Website: www.micromedical.co.uk

Vitalograph Ltd

Maids Moreton
Buckingham MK18 1SW
Tel: 01280 827110
Website: www.vitalograph.co.uk

BREATHLESSNESS QUESTIONNAIRES AVAILABLE

Breathing Problems Questionnaire

Professor Michael Hyland
Department of Psychology

University of Plymouth
Devon PL4 8AA
Email: mhyland@plymouth.ac.uk

Chronic Respiratory Disease Index Questionnaire

Peggy Austin and Dr H Schünemann
Room 2C12
McMaster University Health
Sciences Centre
Hamilton
Ontario
Canada L8N 3Z5
Email: austinp@mcmaster.ca or schuneh@mcmaster.ca

St George's Respiratory Questionnaire

Professor Paul Jones
Division of Physiological Medicine
St Georges Hospital Medical School
Cranmer Terrace
London SW17 0RE
Email: sadie@sghms.ac.uk

GSK

GlaxoSmithKline
Stockley Park West
Uxbridge
Middlesex UB11 1BT
Tel: 0800 221 441
Website: www.customercontactuk@gsk.com

Index